HJH P
(Hub)

Communicating Health

*An action guide to health education
and health promotion*

John Hubley

MACMILLAN

First published 1993 by
MACMILLAN EDUCATION LTD
London and Oxford
Companies and representatives throughout the world

www.macmillan-africa.com

ISBN 0–333–57679–9

16	15	14	13	12	11	10	9	8	7
09	08	07	06	05	04	03	02	01	00

This book is printed on paper suitable for recycling and
made from fully managed and sustained forest sources.

Printed in China

A catalogue record for this book is available from the
British Library.

TALC received assistance in the production of this book as a low-cost
edition from the Swedish International Development Authority.

Contents

Introduction

Malnutrition and infectious disease lead to a heavy burden of sickness and death in developing countries. In addition, most developing countries are experiencing considerable social change with changing family structures, urbanization and adoption of Western lifestyles including diet, smoking, alcohol and drugs. The prevention of disease and the promotion of health lie not in the hands of the medical profession and doctors but in the lifestyles and social conditions in which people live.

This book is aimed at those of you who find yourselves in a position where you are having to plan programmes to improve the health of your communities. I hope to present you with a 'state of the art' view of the best of what is currently practised in developing countries as well as approaches from industrialized countries. While a great deal is talked about health education and health promotion, they are often poorly understood and not done very well. In this book I have tried to explore some of the reasons for which health education programmes have failed in the past and provide practical guidelines for strengthening communication components of your health education and health promotion programmes.

The overall structure of the book is shown on page viii. Chapter 1 provides an introduction to health education and health promotion and Chapters 2–4 act as core chapters. Further details of particular methods are given in Chapters 5–10 and the final chapter provides guidelines on planning, evaluation and implementation. You should look upon the content of this book as guidelines rather than a set of rules. What may work in one community may not work in another. But if you apply these methods in a systematic way, involve the communities you are working with, evaluate and learn from mistakes, you should be able to improve the effectiveness of your activities.

The amount of information that can be provided in a book of this length is inevitably limited. For those wishing to read further, I have prepared an appendix with a list of readily available books, most of which are supplied by Teaching Aids at Low Cost. Health education and health promotion are fast-moving subjects. To help you follow these I have given details of newsletters and journals, many of which are free to persons from developing countries. I have also provided addresses of resource agencies who might be able to help you in your work. I would be happy to hear from you about the work you are doing and receive comments on this book. Good luck in your work!

Dr John Hubley

Introducing health education and health promotion	*basic concepts*

Understanding behaviour The communication process The effective teacher	*core theory*

Face-to-face Working with communities Communication – the people's way! Using media Working with children and young people Politics and health	*specific methods*

Putting it into practice (Programme planning and management)	*implementation*

Acknowledgements

I would like to acknowledge the ideas and support received from a number of persons: the students on the various health education courses I have taught and learned so much from at Leeds and on the various workshops I have facilitated in other countries; my colleagues at Leeds who have provided so much stimulation and ideas, especially June Copeman, John Mee, Maggie Holt, Iona Gordon, Keith Tones and Peter Cox.

I would also like to acknowledge the inspiration and stimulation provided by Professor David Morley and Dr Felicity Savage King whose encouragement was so important at the early stages of preparing this book.

This book is dedicated to the memory of Vikasbhai, Harry Dickinson and Ken Cripwell. In their different ways all three had significant influence on my thinking about health and development and their untimely deaths were a great loss.

I would like to thank the various health educators with whom I have had the privilege of working or exchanging ideas, including: Professor Joshua Adeniyi, Marieke Boot, Dr Bill Brieger, Ann Burgess, Dr Ben Chirwa, Susan Durston, Jane Bunnaq Haile, Dr Saroj Jha, Glenn Laverack, George McBean, Dr Chandra Mouli, Pitnera Mthembu, Nilanjana Mukerji, Martha Osei, Dr Kathy Parker, Jean Ritchie, Mary Roodkowsky, Devi Srestha, David Werner and Cathy Wolfheim.

While many of the ideas in this book were obtained while working as consultant in Africa, the Caribbean, Asia and the Pacific for WHO, UNICEF, the EC and the Overseas Development Agency, the ideas in this book do not represent the views of any of these agencies. The responsibility for any mistakes or inaccuracies is entirely my own.

And finally, thanks to Penny, Alice and Caroline Hubley for their continued support, patience and tolerance during the course of writing this book and my long absences.

Illustrations and photographs

Grateful acknowledgement is made to: WHO South East Asia Region for permission to use illustrations from their manual *Achieving Success in Water and Sanitation*; Ministry of Health, Republic of Fiji for use of illustrations from their *Handbook on Health*; WHO CDD programme for illustration from the *Communication Manager's Guide*; WHO for illustration on patient education and immunization; ARHTAG for permission to use illustrations by Paul Cook on programme-planning; UNICEF in Nepal for use of illustrations from their visual literacy studies and handbook of illustrations and fortune-teller's card; UNICEF EAPRO Regional Headquarters in Bangkok for permission to use cartoons; *Action* comic; Pitnera Mthembu, Ministry of Health, Swaziland; Ministry of Health, Sri Lanka, for leaflet; Dr Patrick Johnson of the Population Communication Institute, Johns Hopkins Institute for photograph of Tatiana and Johnny; Professor David Morley for several illustrations and from *My Name is Today* and *Paediatric*

Priorities; Hermione Lovell for the illustration on the research process; Child to Child for use of the illustration from *Toys for Fun*; John Pinfold and the Leeds University Thailand Hygiene Education Project for reproduction of a page of their storybook on hygiene; International Planned Parenthood for several illustrations.

Every attempt has been made to trace and acknowledge the copyright owners of the illustrations in this book. If a mistake has been made please accept our apologies and we will make due amendments in a future printing.

The photographs are by the author with grateful thanks to the persons who appear in the photographs.

1. Introducing health education and health promotion

We must recognize that most of the world's major health problems and premature deaths are preventable through changes in human behaviour and at low cost. We have the know-how and technology but they have to be transformed into effective action at the community level.

Dr Hiroshi Nakajima, Director-General, World Health Organization, 1988

The aims of this chapter

A starting point for our look at health education and health promotion is the recognition that widespread disease represents a major cause of death, suffering and an obstacle to achieving health. This chapter will consider the following questions.

1. What are the main health problems in developing countries, and their contributory causes?
2. What do we mean by health education and health promotion and why are they important in the prevention of disease and the promotion of health?
3. What is the role of communication in supporting health promotion and health education?
4. What decisions do we have to make to plan and implement effective health education and health promotion programmes in our communities?

Health problems in developing countries

Children at risk

WHO estimates that every year 50 million people die from disease and other causes. Of the total deaths 30 per cent are children under the age of five, most of whom die before their first birthday. Ninety-seven per cent of all infant deaths are in the developing world, where one child in 12 dies before reaching the age of one.

More than half the population in most developing countries are children. The main causes of death in this age group are malnutrition, diarrhoea and respiratory infections. The accumulated burden of low birth-weight, malnutrition, diarrhoea, respiratory and other infections can result in death, stunting and failure to achieve mental and physical potential. This represents a tragic waste – *and most of the causes of death and disability can be prevented*.

Dangerous childbirth

Over half a million women in developing countries die each year from causes related to pregnancy and childbirth, leaving at least one million children motherless. In the poorest countries, the risk of dying from pregnancy and childbirth is 200 times higher than in developed countries. The reasons for maternal mortality are: high number of pregnancies, close spacing of births, lack of ante-natal care,

1

Priority health measures in Third World countries

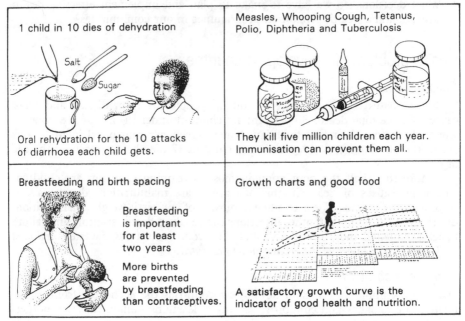

1 child in 10 dies of dehydration

Salt
Sugar

Oral rehydration for the 10 attacks of diarrhoea each child gets.

Measles, Whooping Cough, Tetanus, Polio, Diphtheria and Tuberculosis

They kill five million children each year. Immunisation can prevent them all.

Breastfeeding and birth spacing

Breastfeeding is important for at least two years

More births are prevented by breastfeeding than contraceptives.

Growth charts and good food

A satisfactory growth curve is the indicator of good health and nutrition.

Fig. 1.1 Children are the priority group for health programmes in developing countries

2

lack of access to family planning, unsafe abortion practices and teenage pregnancies. In response to these problems WHO has launched a 'Safe Motherhood Programme'.

Water-related disease

The World Health Organization estimates that 80 per cent of all sickness in the world is due to poor water and sanitation. Five million children die each year from diarrhoea. The Water and Sanitation for Health Project (WASH) in the United States has provided the following figures for the global impact of water-related diseases:

- *Diarrhoeal diseases*: 875 million cases a year;
- *Ascariasis* (roundworms): 900 million cases a year (20 000 end in death);
- *Trachoma*: 500 million cases a year (8 million end in blindness);
- *Hookworm*: 800 million cases a year;
- *Schistosomiasis*: 200 million cases a year;
- *Guinea worm*: 4 million cases a year.
- The daily task of collecting water represents a heavy burden on the women in developing countries, affecting their own health as well as their ability to care for their families.

According to Bradley's environmental classification of water-related diseases, some of these infections are passed through drinking water as *water-borne diseases*. However, many are transmitted through contamination during collection and storage of the water as well as contamination of hands, fingers and food. As water for practising hygiene is often the limiting factor, these are called *water-washed diseases*. In *water-based diseases* such as schistosomiasis, part of the parasite life-cycle is in water. In the *water-related insect vector* diseases such as malaria, onchocerciasis and filariasis, transmission of disease is by an insect that breeds in water.

Fig. 1.2 The World Health Organization estimates that 80 per cent of all sickness is linked to water and sanitation

3

Disability

One in ten persons in the world suffers from some form of disability such as blindness, physical impairment or injuries, resulting in loss of earning and discrimination. It was the International Year of the Disabled in 1981 that first directed attention at the global level to the issue of disability and sought to promote 'full participation and equality of disabled people in all aspects of society and greater public awareness of the needs of disabled people'.

Infectious and parasitic diseases

In developing countries the main disease burden comes from acute infectious diseases and malnutrition. In addition to the water-related diseases described above:

- nearly three million people die each year from tuberculosis – most of which are in the developing world;
- it is possible to immunize against many infectious diseases including measles, polio, pertussis, rubella, tuberculosis and tetanus. WHO estimates that more than 8000 children die each day because they are not immunized against vaccine-preventable diseases. Measles alone kills 1.4 million infants and tetanus kills 767 000 new-borns a year.

AIDS and other sexually-transmitted diseases

AIDS is an example of an infectious disease that is transmitted through sexual intercourse, blood products and from mother to child. It is important to distinguish persons who are infected with the virus but show no symptoms (HIV antibody positive) from those who have developed symptoms of AIDS. AIDS affects both developing and industrialized countries. However, economic difficulties and weaker health care infra-structure will make it difficult for developing countries to mount effective prevention and control programmes for AIDS. The World Health Organization estimates that:

- By 1991 more than 10 million children in Africa may be orphaned through death of parents from AIDS, and family support systems will be inadequate to cope with the scale of the problem.
- The AIDS epidemic in Asia is at an early stage, with a conservative estimate of 1 000 000 persons infected in 1991, mainly in India and Thailand. However, the rapid increase in the number of cases in India and Thailand shows the possible future scale of the problem.
- By the year 2000, based on data as of June 1991, there is likely to be a cumulative world total of:
    25–30 million adult HIV infections and 8–10 million adult AIDS cases;
    5–10 million children with HIV infections and 4–8 million cases of children with AIDS; and *90 per cent of these cases of infection and AIDS will be in the developing countries.*

AIDS represents a major global priority for action. Although there is a greater toll of death from other infectious diseases, the AIDS epidemic has certain features that make it special: there is no cure and the level is increasing.

Tobacco-induced diseases

Worldwide, over one billion people now smoke – averaging over ten cigarettes a day. Many traditional forms of tobacco are smoked, such as the bidi leaf cigarettes in India. More and more people are switching to cigarettes, which account for about 75 per cent of all tobacco consumed.

4

Tobacco affects health in many ways; through nicotine, tar and the effect of the carbon monoxide in the smoke on the body function. The harmful effect of tobacco can be reduced but not eliminated by an effective filter (many of the 'filtered' brands do not have very effective filters) or the smoking of 'low tar' brands.

The health risks of tobacco include: greater likelihood of suffering from some diseases including lung cancer, heart disease and respiratory disorders. Furthermore recent evidence highlights the effect of *passive smoking* – the harmful effects of cigarette smoke breathed in by non-smokers.

Cigarette sales in developing countries are growing at least three times faster than in other countries. The former consume between one-third to over one-half the world's tobacco. Young people in particular are taking up the habit. In Pakistan, cigarette consumption has been growing 8 per cent a year. And the incidence of lung cancer has increased from only 4 per cent to as much as 20 per cent of all new cancers during that same period.

- In Bangladesh the money spent on just five cigarettes a day could pay for one-quarter of a child's daily food needs.
- The firewood used in curing tobacco worldwide is equivalent to 7 million acres of land each year.
- 0.3 per cent of the world's farming land is used for tobacco – enough to feed 10.2 million people if the same land was used for grain.

The new health problems

In addition to tobacco, developing countries are taking up other health problems of industrialized countries – where non-communicable diseases make up 70–80

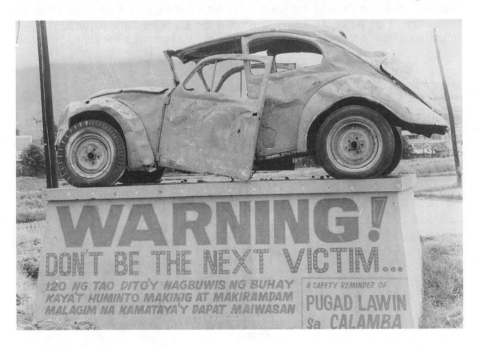

Fig. 1.3 Social changes in the developing countries are leading to new health problems such as traffic accidents

per cent of all deaths. Part of the reason for this shift can be explained simply by the fact that, as conditions improve, people are living longer and there are more chronic diseases such as heart disease and cancers. However, other reasons are the dramatic social changes taking place in developing countries:

- increased numbers of elderly persons in the population requiring care and support;
- expansion of cities and urban living resulting in greater mobility, separation of families and removal of traditional systems of support, and poor housing;
- increased industrialization resulting in pollution and occupational diseases, including accidents, exposure to harmful dust, chemicals and noise;
- more motor cars and traffic, leading to increase in deaths from road traffic accidents;
- sexually-transmitted diseases and AIDS encouraged by changing patterns of sexual behaviour, breaking up of family structures, growth of sex tourism;
- changes in diet, especially sugar, fat and salt, resulting in increase in dental decay, obesity, heart disease, hypertension, diabetes, cancer of the bowel, appendicitis – the 'diseases of westernization' (WHO estimates that at least half of all deaths from cardio-vascular diseases can be prevented);
- greater availability of addictive substances including tobacco, alcohol and drugs;
- conflicts of commercial interests and health – the damage done by advertising and promotion of tobacco, baby milk, cigarettes and inappropriate medicines.

Influences on health

In order to decide what actions are needed to prevent disease and promote health we need to be able to identify influences on health. In particular, we need to be able to distinguish those about which very little can be done from others that we *can* change. One factor we cannot control is the genes we have acquired through inheritance from our parents. For example, a person born with the genetic disorder

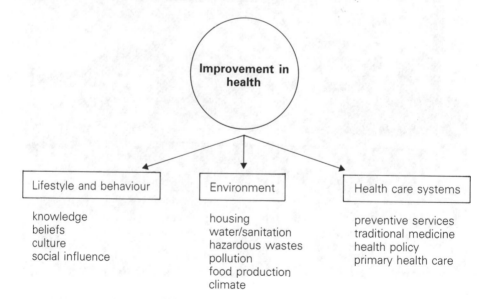

Fig. 1.4 Influences on health

sickle-cell anaemia has the disease for life and should receive counselling to help them to cope with it. The influences of climate, geography and genetic inheritance that we cannot change are sometimes called non-behavioural.

But many causes of disease can be changed. To prevent disease we must concentrate on those causes that we can change and these are the factors to which we must devote our attention.

There are other ways of looking at influences. Later in this chapter you will see how it is possible to consider the *level of influence* – whether the factors that influence health are under the individual's control or operate at the family, community, district, national or international level. Another approach is to separate out those influences that are *cultural*.

One approach that I have found useful is given in Figure 1.4 which is adapted from the *Health Field Model* used by the Canadian Government in their influential policy document 'The Health of the Canadians'. As a practical model, it separates the influences into three inter-related areas: those due to behaviour or 'lifestyle'; those that can be influenced by improved health care systems; and those that are determined by the environment.

Environment

The environment, especially climate, has an important influence on our health. Disease, food production and access to drinking water are influenced by temperature, rainfall, soil conditions and vegetation. Diseases such as diarrhoea and malaria have a higher incidence in the rainy season. Deserts, forests, swamps and coastal regions will all affect the health of their communities.

Although the environment has a profound effect on health, its effects are linked to other factors, especially the behaviour and action of people. For example, building dams, irrigation projects, cutting forests, over-grazing of land by animals, factory pollution and wars can all affect the environment and health. Even so-called 'natural' disasters such as earthquakes, volcanic eruptions, hurricanes and cyclones raise important questions about human behaviour and social forces. What conditions make people live in disaster-prone areas? Why cannot the poor afford to build houses strong enough to resist earthquakes?

The contribution of health services to health

In recent years more and more people are asking the question: *do health services make people healthy?* In most countries, too much emphasis is put on treatment rather than prevention, urban rather than rural health and meeting the health needs of the richer sections of the community rather than those of the poor.

Many countries, on achieving independence, copied health care systems in Europe and the USA, with their emphasis on curative care based on doctors, drugs and hospitals. However, it is increasingly being realized that the promotion of health and the prevention of disease do not lie in large hospitals.

The introduction of the concept of *Primary Health Care* by the World Health Assembly in the Russian city of Alma Ata in 1978 was a direct result of the failure of curative hospital-based systems of health care. It was realized that most of the important health problems in the world can be dealt with by a combination of decentralized basic health care and prevention. The *Alma Ata Declaration* went on to say:

Primary health care is essential health care based on practical, scientifically sound and socially acceptable methods and technology made universally accessible to individuals and families in the community through their full participation and at a cost that the community and country can afford to maintain at every stage of their development in the spirit of self-reliance and self-determination.

The full text of the Alma Ata Declaration is a remarkable document that emphasizes the importance of preventive measures including provision of food, housing, water, sanitation and health education. It also clearly states that improvement of health cannot be separated from discussions about social concerns such as poverty and social justice.

The idea of primary health care does not ignore the significant role that medicine can make to improvement of health. Health services should be *appropriate* – effective, affordable and acceptable to the communities. When you are considering a health issue such as a cholera outbreak, diarrhoea, lung cancer or

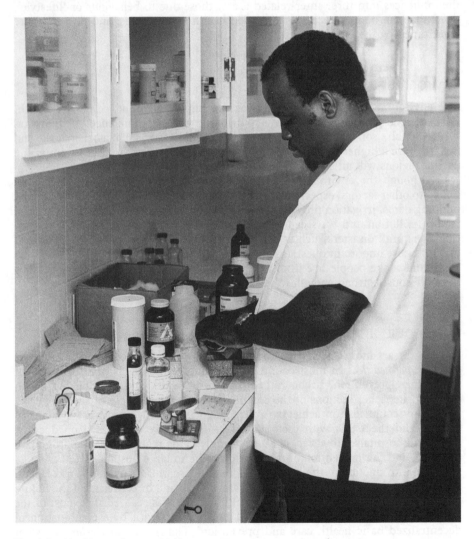

Fig. 1.5 Health services on their own cannot prevent disease and promote health

maternal health there are some fundamental questions that you should ask, to decide what role, if any, health services can play:

- How good is our current understanding about the health topic? Can it be prevented? Is there a vaccine available? Can we screen people at risk or at early stages of the disease?
- What, if any, health services are necessary for prevention?
- How effective are home remedies and traditional medicines?
- Can it be cured? Are drugs available?
- If the disease cannot be cured, what can be done to make the condition of the patient as comfortable as possible?
- What kinds of health services are needed for treatment and care at lowest cost to the community?

Human behaviour

Most health issues cannot be dealt with by drugs and treatment alone. The promotion of health and prevention of disease will usually involve some changes in lifestyles or human behaviour. There can be confusion over terms used.

- The words *actions, practices* and *behaviours* are different words for the same thing.
- *Lifestyle* refers to the collection of behaviours that make up a person's way of life – including diet, clothing, family life, housing and work.
- *Customs* are behaviours that are shared by many people.
- *Traditions* are behaviours that have been carried out for a long time and handed down from parents to children.

Here are listed some of the many kinds of behaviours that have an influence on health, and the ten key behaviours for improvement of child health that UNICEF, WHO and UNESCO identified in their initiative *Facts for Life*.

Examples of behaviours promoting health and preventing disease

---

Health behaviours: actions that healthy people undertake to keep themselves or others healthy and prevent disease, e.g. exercise, good nutrition, breast-feeding, weaning, latrines, child-spacing, hygiene practices, tooth-brushing, taking anti-malaria drugs; reduction of health-damaging behaviours, such as smoking, bottlefeeding, excessive alcohol consumption and accidents. These behaviours may be based on decisions or are done regularly and have become habits – or routines.

Utilization behaviours: utilization of health services, such as ante-natal, child health, immunization, family-planning and screening programmes.

Illness behaviours: recognition of early symptoms and prompt self-referral for treatment, such as oral rehydration.

Compliance behaviours: following a course of prescribed drugs, such as for tuberculosis.

Rehabilitation behaviours: what people need to do after a serious illness to prevent further disability.

Community action: actions by individuals and groups to change and improve their surroundings to meet special needs.

---

1. The health of both women and children can be significantly improved by spacing births at least two years apart, by avoiding pregnancies before the age of 18 and by limiting the total number of pregnancies to four.
2. To reduce the dangers of childbearing, all pregnant women should go to a health worker for pre-natal care and all births should be assisted by a trained person.
3. For the first few months of a baby's life, breastmilk *alone* is the best possible food and drink. Infants need other foods, in addition to breastmilk, when they are four-to-six months old.
4. Children under three have special feeding needs. They need to eat five or six times a day and their food should be specially enriched by adding mashed vegetables and small amounts of fats or oils.
5. Diarrhoea can kill by draining too much liquid from a child's body. So the liquid lost each time the child passes a watery stool must be replaced by giving the child plenty of the right liquids to drink – breastmilk, diluted gruel, soup, or a special drink called Oral Rehydration Solution (ORS). If the illness is more serious than usual, the child needs help from a health worker and the special ORS drink. A child with diarrhoea also needs food to make a good recovery.
6. Immunization protects against several diseases which can cause poor growth, disability and death. All immunizations should be completed in the first year of the child's life. Every woman of childbearing age should be immunized against tetanus.
7. Most coughs and colds will get better on their own. But if a child with a cough is breathing much more rapidly than normal, then the child is seriously ill and it is essential to go to a health centre quickly. A child with a cough or cold should be helped to eat and to drink plenty of liquids.
8. Many illnesses are caused because germs enter the mouth. This can be prevented by using latrines; by washing hands with soap and water after using the latrine and before handling food; by keeping food and water clean and by boiling drinking water if it is not from a safe piped supply.
9. Illnesses hold back a child's growth. After an illness, a child needs an extra meal every day for a week to make up the growth lost.
10. Children between the ages of six months and three years should be weighed every month. If there is no gain in weight for two months, something is wrong.

The role of human behaviour in prevention of disease

There are three levels of prevention (see Figure 1.6).

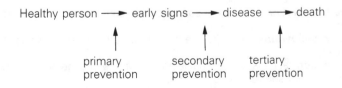

Fig. 1.6 Levels of prevention of disease

Primary prevention

Primary prevention consists of all those activities carried out to keep healthy people healthy and prevent them getting disease.

Secondary prevention

Secondary prevention is the name given to interventions at the early stage of a problem before it becomes serious. It is important to ensure that the community can recognize early signs of disease and go for treatment before the disease becomes serious. Health problems such as leprosy and tuberculosis can be cured if the disease is caught at an early stage. The actions people take before consulting a health care worker, including recognition of symptoms, taking home remedies ('self-medication'), consulting family and healers are called *illness behaviours* and are shown in Figure 1.7.

Fig. 1.7 Stages in illness behaviour

Screening is the name given to the process of surveying a community with tests to detect diseases at an early stage before people feel symptoms. A good example of this is the cervical smear test which detects unusual 'pre-cancerous' cells in a woman's cervix before they develop into cancer. Another example of screening is growth-monitoring of young children. If a child is regularly weighed and the weights are plotted on a growth chart, you can see from the chart if there is a slowing-down of growth. Advice can then be given to the parents to prevent the child becoming malnourished. Although screening is carried out by health services, educational programmes are still needed to encourage people to come forward for screening.

It is better to prevent disease. But people will still get sick and need treatment. Even at this stage actions and behaviours of the patient are essential to getting well again. Tertiary prevention overlaps with secondary prevention and includes behaviours that are involved in treatment and rehabilitation.

Recovery from treatment and operations may involve some rehabilitation programmes. For example, after a period in bed, a person may need physiotherapy and exercise to recover full strength. Help is needed to help a person adjust to artificial limbs or using a wheelchair. The rehabilitation process can involve meeting both a person's physical and psychological needs.

An important part of tertiary prevention is to ensure patients *follow treatment procedures*: if patients are prescribed medicines, it is essential that they take them correctly. The health worker must explain when to take them, for how long and what to do if there are any side-effects.

Tuberculosis is a good example of the importance of following treatment procedures. The drugs for treatment of tuberculosis are effective but require taking regularly over a period of one or two years. People often mistakenly believe that they are cured once they feel better, stop taking the drug, and experience a relapse of tuberculosis.

Doctors may prescribe unnecessary drugs and patients sometimes insist on being given a medicine. For example, many children with diarrhoea are prescribed antibiotics which are not effective against most childhood diarrhoea and delay the life-saving oral rehydration. The overuse of medicine can be an expensive drain on the budget of the family and the health services as well as encouraging the development of antibody-resistant bacteria. WHO has launched an essential drugs programme that identifies the most important drugs that are needed to meet most common diseases at the cheapest cost. Control of advertising by commercial drug companies, training of doctors and education of the public are all needed to reduce the amount of unnecessary prescribing of drugs.

However, the real danger of unnecessary use of medicines is not the one of cost, but that it encourages the belief that achievement of health lies only in medicines. It draws attention away from the need for actions by governments and individuals to improve living conditions and encourage health-promoting behaviours.

Behavioural diagnosis

The term behavioural diagnosis is used to describe the process by which we look at the causes of health problems and find out whether human behaviour is involved – either in prevention or treatment. In the behavioural diagnosis we list all the behaviours that the community should carry out for primary, secondary and tertiary prevention of the disease. It is the behaviours of the persons *themselves* in the community that are identified. Later in the planning stage you will have to consider what determines these behaviours; especially the role of social and economic factors such as poverty, inequalities, inappropriate health services and government policies.

The key messages in 'Facts for Life' are an example of the behavioural diagnosis applied to a general health topic – child health. We can also apply the concept of behavioural diagnosis to general programme areas such as water and sanitation. The role of health education and communication support in promoting uptake of water and sanitation technologies and achieving health benefits is as shown in the list.

community participation in the installation of improved water supply;
use and maintenance of improved water supplies including avoidance of unimproved
sources, clean collection and storage of water in the home;
building of latrines and upgrading of unimproved latrines to improve them;
correct use of latrines, especially by groups such as children;
maintaining the new improved latrines;
hygiene practices, especially washing of hands with soap after use of latrines and
before preparation of food and eating; clean storage of food and utensils; personal
hygiene, washing of children and babies; washing of clothing; disposal of dirty water
from washing, etc.

Our changing knowledge

There are many examples where health educators have wasted time and effort persuading people to adopt practices that were later found not to be relevant. For example, in the 1980s many health workers mistakenly encouraged mothers to give high-protein foods to children to prevent the form of malnutrition called kwashiorkor. We now know that lack of protein foods in the diet is not a direct cause of kwashiorkor and nutritionists emphasize adding oils/fats to weaning diets to enrich the energy content.

Although our understanding of health and disease is improving, many field-workers are still using out-of-date and inaccurate information in their health education. Even the so-called 'experts' do not always agree. The public can get very confused with conflicting messages and do not know which to follow. It is not surprising that they often become impatient and ignore us!

It was in response to this need to avoid confusion that the 'Facts for Life' campaign was launched. But, as knowledge improves, you should continually expect changes in the future. A good way for you to keep up with new developments is to put yourself on the mailing list of the free newsletters produced by international agencies (see Appendix B).

The need to understand human behaviour

It is a common complaint that the community ignore advice and continue to practise health-damaging behaviours even when they know them to be harmful. It is easy to condemn the community and put the blame on traditional beliefs or backwardness. The real reason for failure, however, is often that the health education does not take into account the underlying influences on health, contains irrelevant information, promotes unrealistic changes, is directed at the wrong people and uses inappropriate methods. So, to promote health, it is important to determine the factors that underlie a person's decision to perform or not perform a behaviour.

Human behaviour plays an important role in the prevention, control, treatment and rehabilitation processes of most health problems. However, Figure 1.8 shows that the influences on a person's behaviour may be outside their control at the family, community, district, national and even international level.

Individual	Community		National	
beliefs ⎱ values ⎬ of individual attitudes ⎰ person only	beliefs ⎱ values ⎬ attitudes ⎰	shared by whole community	beliefs ⎱ values ⎬ attitudes ⎰	shared by whole nation
susceptibility to pressure from family and community	influence of community leaders, elders and opinion leaders (norms)		mass media advertising and marketing by commercial companies	
knowledge, skills and education	quantity, quality and appropriateness of local services: health, education		government policies on education and agriculture, etc.	
genetic endowment	agriculture and sanitation etc.		national health education services	
economic situation of individual and family	socio-economic condition of community		socio-economic condition of country	

Fig. 1.8 Individual, community and national levels of influence on health

Some problems, like lack of water, are too big to be tackled by individual families. The whole community must act together to deal with these. So in looking at the influences on a behaviour we may decide that the change must take place at the level of the whole community. Our understanding of behaviour may show that there are many influences outside the individual's control that are actually *damaging* health. These outside influences could include advertising health-damaging products such as cigarettes or baby foods, government policies such as promoting tobacco cultivation or location of health services, poverty and unemployment. *Victim-blaming is the name given to the process when poorly-planned health education directs itself at changing the individual and ignores the factors outside the individual that influence behaviour.*

Health promotion

Many feel that too much effort has been placed on programmes aimed at individuals. They have pointed to the importance of working with communities to influence economic and political factors at the community or national level. They have stressed the need to persuade governments to pass health-promoting laws, such as control of advertising of tobacco and baby foods, and supporting the expansion of primary health care programmes and agricultural development.

The term *health promotion* is increasingly being used to draw attention to the need for both educational and political action to influence health. At a meeting in Canada in 1986, the Ottawa Charter on Health Promotion was drawn up. This conference mainly focused on the needs in industrialized countries, but also took into account similar concerns in other regions. The Charter emphasized that promoting health is more than just providing health services. Peace, housing, education, food, income, a sustainable environment, social justice and equity are all necessary for achievement of health. It calls for people to act as *advocates* for health through the addressing of political, economic, social, cultural, environmental, behavioural and biological factors.

Extracts from the Ottawa Charter on Health Promotion

Health promotion is the process of enabling people to increase control over, and to improve, their health. To reach a state of complete physical, mental and social well-being, an individual or group must be able to identify and to realize aspirations, to satisfy needs, and to change or cope with the environment. Health is, therefore, seen as a resource for everyday life, not the objective of living. Health is a positive concept emphasizing social and personal resources, as well as physical capacities. Therefore, health promotion is not just the responsibility of the health sector, but goes beyond healthy life-styles to well-being.

HEALTH PROMOTION ACTION MEANS:

Building healthy public policy Health promotion goes beyond health care. It puts health on the agenda of policy makers in all sectors and at all levels. It directs policy makers to be aware of the health consequences of their decisions and to accept their responsibilities for health.

Health promotion policy combines diverse but complementary approaches including legislation, fiscal measures, taxation and organizational change. It is coordinated action that leads to health, income and social policies that foster greater equity. Joint action contributes to ensuring safer and healthier goods and services healthier public services, and cleaner, more enjoyable environments.

Health-promotion policy requires the identification of obstacles to the adoption of healthy public policies in non-health sectors, and ways of removing them. The aim must be to make the healthier choice the easier choice.

Creating supportive environments Health promotion generates living and working conditions that are safe, stimulating, satisfying and enjoyable. Systematic assessment of the health impact of a rapidly changing environment – particularly in areas of technology, work, energy production and urbanization – is essential and must be followed by action to ensure positive benefit to the health of the public. The protection of the natural and built environments and the conservation of natural resources must be addressed in any health promotion strategy.

Strengthening community action At the heart of this process is the empowerment of communities, their ownership and control of their own endeavours and destinies. Community development draws on existing human and material resources in the community to enhance self-help and social support, and to develop flexible systems for strengthening public participation and direction of health matters.

Developing personal skills Health promotion supports personal and social development through providing information, education for health and enhancing life skills. By so doing, it increases the options available to people to exercise more control over their health and environment, and to make choices conducive to health. Enabling people to learn throughout life, to prepare themselves for all of its stages and to cope with chronic illness and injuries is essential. This has to be facilitated in school, home, work and community settings. Action is required through educational, professional, commercial and voluntary bodies, and within the institutions themselves.

Reorienting health services The responsibility for health promotion in health services is shared among individuals, community groups, health professionals, health service institutions and governments. They must work together towards a health care system that contributes to the pursuit of health. Reorienting health services also requires stronger attention to health research as well as changes in professional education and training. This must lead to a change of attitude and organization of health services, which refocuses on the total needs of the individual as a whole person.

Ethics of health promotion and behaviour change

Most health promotion programmes seek to influence families, the community and decision-makers to make changes, either in their own lives, or in policies that affect other people's health. This raises important questions about the ethics of behaviour-change. Look at the questions below. How would you answer them?

- Is it right for health promotors to persuade or pass laws to try to influence people to change their behaviour?
- Under what conditions do you think it might be justified to try to make someone do something that they do not want to do?
- When do you think it is better to leave the persons themselves to make the decision as to the behaviour change?
- Can people living in a state of poverty and oppression make decisions and control their own lives?

These questions pose important *ethical* issues. Some people argue that individuals should have the right to do what they want to do and that we should not interfere. This is a common response when we try to persuade smokers to give up smoking.

But should a person have the freedom to choose, if their actions may also harm others? For example a person who smokes is not only damaging his or her own health but also others who breathe in the smoke – for example, their children. Someone who drinks alcohol while driving can endanger other people's lives. A food-handler has a responsibility to practise good hygiene to preserve the health of those who consume the food. Public health often involves restricting the behaviour of individuals for the good of the community. However, the decisions on what should be changed are not only medical ones – but involve social, religious and moral considerations.

Some people argue that the community should be left to make its own decisions. However the community may have an incomplete understanding of health and diseases: they may not be aware of the existence of innovations such as immunization, oral rehydration therapy or improved pit-latrines. Failure to tell the community about these life-saving new practices might also be considered unethical.

Health education

Information and education provide the informed base for making choices. They are necessary and core components of health promotion, which aims at **increasing knowledge and disseminating information** related to health. This should include: the public's perceptions and experiences of health and how it might be sought; knowledge from epidemiology, social and other sciences on the patterns of health and disease and factors affecting them; and descriptions of the 'total' environment in which health and health choices are shaped.

(WHO Policy Statement on Health Promotion)

Health education is one of the most important components of health promotion and involves a combination of the following:

- motivation to adopt health-promoting behaviours;
- helping people to make decisions about their health and acquire the necessary confidence and skills to put their decisions into practice.

The concept of human behaviour is emphasized by the American health educator Lawrence Green who defines health education as 'any combination of learning opportunities designed to facilitate voluntary adaptation of behaviour which will improve or maintain health'. The use of the word 'voluntary' is significant for ethical reasons. It implies that health educators should not force people to do what they do not want to do. Instead our efforts should help people to make decisions and choices for themselves.

Helen Ross and Paul Mico have provided another useful definition of health education: 'A process with intellectual, psychological and social dimensions relating to activities that increase the abilities of people to make informed decisions affecting their personal, family and community well-being. This process, based on scientific principles, facilitates learning and behavioural change in both health personnel and consumers, including children and youth.' The term health education will be used throughout this book to cover health education and broadly similar activities carried out under different names. Some alternative terms in the list are equivalent to health education, others are based on narrower approaches and assumptions.

Various terms used for communication and health education activities

---

Information, education and communication (IEC) is a term originally from family planning and more recently AIDS control programmes in developing countries. It is increasingly being used as a general term for communication activities to promote health.

Communication support is a term for describing support programmes for introduction of water, sanitation and hygiene education. Heili Perret has defined communication support as 'Information, motivation and education activities which are specifically designed to encourage the participation of intended beneficiaries in a project and to improve the project's impact on development'.

Social marketing involves the application of commercial marketing and advertising approaches to health and has been used for promotion of condoms and oral rehydration solution.

Social mobilization is a term now popular with UNICEF to describe a campaign approach combining mass media and working with community groups and organizations.

Extension comes originally from the agricultural extension approach of promoting change through demonstrations, working with opinion leaders and community-based educational activities.

Nutrition education is education directed at the promotion of nutrition and covers choice of food, food-preparation and storage of food.

Population education includes education on family planning; 'family life education' is another related term for education of young people in a range of topics that include family planning, child rearing and child care and responsible parenthood.

Patient-education is a term for education in hospital and clinic settings linked to following of treatment procedures, medication, home care and rehabilitation procedures.

Other 'education' activities Antenatal education, AIDS education, dental health education and mental health education are all specialized areas of health education.

Communication in health education and health promotion

In its simplest form, communication involves exchanges of information between people. Most educational activities involve communication of some kind or other. Chapter 3 discusses the different ways that communication can happen and the psychological processes involved. As shown in Figure 1.9, communication is an essential part of *all* health promotion activities in order to:

- have a dialogue with communities including minorities and disadvantaged groups;
- influence decision-makers to adopt health promoting policies and laws;
- raise awareness among decision-makers of issues of poverty, human rights, equity, environmental issues;
- ensure that the public gives support to government health-promoting policies;
- communicate new laws and policies to the public;
- raise public awareness of issues in order to mobilize community participation;
- develop community action on health issues.

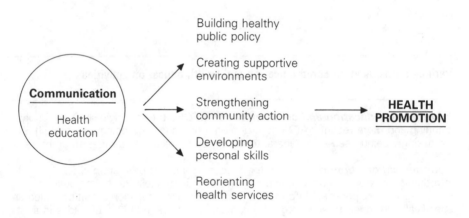

Fig. 1.9 Communication and health promotion

What approach to use?

Even if the main aim of health education is to influence behaviour, there is still a range of possible approaches that might include:

- the ***persuasion approach*** – the deliberate attempt to influence the other person to do what we want them to do (often called the 'directive' approach or, when done forcefully, coercion);
- the ***informed decision-making approach*** – giving people information, problem-solving and decision-making skills to make decisions but leaving the actual choice to the person; with groups who have been disadvantaged and oppressed this can also involve promoting awareness – 'consciousness-raising' – and building confidence that they have the power to make decisions and control their own lives – *empowerment*.

One educationalist who has had a profound influence is Paulo Freire. He was deeply critical of formal 'didactic' approaches to education where the teacher was seen to be the expert passing knowledge to the pupils. In his literacy work among the peasants of northeast Brazil, he pioneered an alternative approach to education called 'conscientization'. His methods aimed to develop critical awareness, raising of consciousness and stimulating people to think how they can change their environment.

Many health educators feel that, instead of using persuasion and coercion, it is better to work with communities to develop their problem-solving skills and provide the information to help them make *informed choices*. However in situations where there is a serious threat such as an epidemic, and the actions needed are clearcut, it might be considered justified to persuade people to adopt specific behaviour changes.

Should you focus on specific diseases or promote health?

You will need to decide whether to focus on prevention of particular diseases, e.g. AIDS, diarrhoea or a broader approach. The advantage of taking a single disease approach is that it is often easier to mobilize the public, other field workers and potential sponsors and workers on a single issue. However, many prefer the broader approach because they feel that it is better to emphasize health and a healthy lifestyle rather than disease. In health care planning, the name given to the approach which focuses on individual diseases is 'vertical' planning; the alternative one of taking a broader health-focused approach is 'horizontal'.

Who should the education be directed at?

An individual's behaviour is extremely important for his or her health. But it is not always the individual who makes the decisions and should be the 'target group'. We often find that a person's behaviour is influenced by other persons in the family and community and these social pressures are examined further in the next chapter. Communications should be directed at the persons who make the key decisions in the family and community – the 'gate keepers'.

Even when you have decided on a particular 'target group' you will need to consider at what point in that person's life is the best time to reach them. We can think of the human lifecycle, or *health career*, as a series of stages from the young child to the school-age child to the adult and the elderly person (Figure 1.10). In the educational diagnosis we must decide at what stage to carry out our health education. A well-planned programme will include educational activities directed at a range of different age groups.

old person

↑

adult

↑

young adult

↑

secondary school

↑

primary school

↑

pre-school child

Fig. 1.10 A 'health career': at what stage in the human life cycle should one intervene?

At what level should the intervention take place?

You could operate your communication activities at a range of levels: the individual, family, community, district, region, national and international. For example you could work with individuals using one-to-one education, you could spend time with the family, mobilize community participation or act at a national level to influence policy.

How you choose the level to operate at will depend on the problems you are facing, the special advantages to be gained from each level and the resources and opportunities that are available to you. Your analysis of the influences on behaviour (see Figure 1.8) might have told you that the important influences that you have to change are at one level, e.g. at the national level. However, if you are based in a local community you may not be able to work at the national level.

What channels can you work through?

You will have to decide on the best way of reaching your intended audience – home, community, clinics, school, workplace, markets, public places, bars or clubs? For example, women of childbearing age can often be reached through child health services, adult men could be reached through the workplace and children through schools. Mass media such as radio would be suitable for reaching the general population, whereas messages for specific groups are best communicated through face-to-face communication.

Decisions are also needed as to *who* will do the communication. Are there people that you can involve in educational activities, such as teachers, youth leaders, employers, politicians, musicians? Health promotion and health education are part of the work of a wide range of persons in health, education, social and other services and they can be mobilized. You might decide to work through non-governmental agencies such as Red Cross, planned parenthood associations, churches, boy scouts or self-help and community-based groups. As part of primary health care activities, many countries have mobilized local volunteers as community health workers and these also provide a valuable resource for health education.

What method will you use for reaching the intended audience?

A further set of choices concerns the educational methods to be used. Earlier decisions on target audiences and channels may have already determined the choice. For example, if you choose to work through schools to reach young people, your methods will probably involve classroom activities, educational projects and field visits. Some of the many different communication methods are shown in Figure 1.12.

Chapter 3 will review some of the advantages and disadvantages of different educational methods and the influence of source, method, channel and receiver on the effectiveness of communication.

What is the best timing for your programme?

You will have to decide on the best timing for your communication activity. An intensive approach for a short time period is called a *campaign*. In a campaign it is often possible to involve a large number of different groups for a short period of intensive activity. For example, campaigns have been used for immunization programmes in Latin America. In Honduras, a campaign using radio and leaflets to promote oral rehydration was held at the start of the rainy season just before the peak period of diarrhoea.

Health services
Doctors and nurses in primary
   health care
midwives
health visitors
public health nurses
village health workers
nutrition programmes
immunization programmes

Public health services
public health inspectors
water supply
sanitation
hygiene inspection
refuse collection

Informal processes in the community
elders
parents and child-rearing
traditional birth attendants
traditional healers
village leaders
religious leaders
non-governmental organizations

Education services
teachers in primary and secondary
   schools
adult education
literacy programmes
pre-school programmes
vocational training

Agriculture and socio-economic development
agricultural extension
community development
applied nutrition programmes
cooperatives
employment-generating programmes
women's programmes

Fig. 1.11   Many people can be mobilized for health education in the community

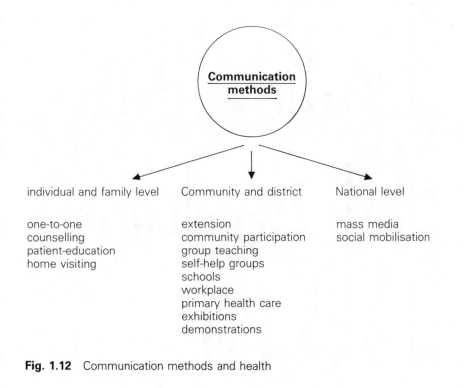

Communication
methods

individual and family level

one-to-one
counselling
patient-education
home visiting

Community and district

extension
community participation
group teaching
self-help groups
schools
workplace
primary health care
exhibitions
demonstrations

National level

mass media
social mobilisation

Fig. 1.12   Communication methods and health

Table 1.1 Key of areas of decision-making in communication and health education

Broad approach	Horizontal or vertical programme	Target groups	Level of operation	Channel or method for reaching target group/strategy	Time scale for activities undertaken
DIRECTIVE	HORIZONTAL	women	individual	health services	SHORT-TERM intensive activity (campaign approach)
agency-determined objectives	general lifestyle improvement	children	family	primary health care services	
specific behavioural outcomes	or	men	community	schools	LONGER TERM approach with greater integration
or	VERTICAL	pregnant women	district	mass media	
PROCESS	nutrition	parents of pre-school children	region	churches	
educational	AIDS	elderly	national	voluntary sector	
empowerment	STDs	teenagers	international	community project	
decision-making	alcohol	schoolchildren		workplace	
participation	tobacco	out-of-school youth		intersectoral collaboration	
	drugs	college students		politicians	
	malaria	healthworkers		self-help groups	
	schistosomiasis	factory workers			
	diarrhoea	politicians			
	cancer	opinion leaders			
	family planning	etc.			
	dental disease				
	immunization				
	etc.				

Some people are critical of the campaign approach because they feel that it is short-lasting. They claim that it is better to develop an 'on-going' programme that is 'institutionalized' into the daily work of services such as clinics, community health services and schools. Others find campaigns useful as a way of generating enthusiasm and involving a wide range of organizations in supporting your work.

Summary

You can see that communication, health education and health promotion should be a component of any programme for improving the health of a community. Without an active communication component, health services will have little impact on people's health.

Table 1.1 summarizes some of these key decisions on approaches described above. Making these decisions will involve adopting a *systematic approach* to planning communication activities. This will involve studying the problem, gathering information on your communities and working out answers to the following questions.

- What is the problem?
- What are the causes of the problem?
- What is the role of human behaviour?
- What is the role of health promotion, including government action, legislation and policymaking in dealing with the problem?
- What is the role of health education and communication?
- Who should the communication and health education be directed at?
- What approach should be used – persuasion or informed decision-making? single issue or broad-based health? intensive campaign or ongoing programme?
- What level (individual, family, community, national, international etc.) should the communication carried out?
- What channel should be used to reach the intended audience?
- What methods should be used?

2. Understanding human behaviour

In Chapter 1 you saw how an important justification for health education and health promotion comes from the fact that health is determined, not by medical services and drugs, but by ordinary human actions and behaviours. Many health education programmes have failed because they neglected to understand the cultural, social, economic and political factors that influence these actions. Some people are critical of studying human behaviour and claim that this puts too much emphasis on individual action rather than the need for political, social and economic change. However, a proper understanding of the influences on human behaviour will avoid the pitfalls of *victim-blaming*. It can do this by separating out those influences that are under the control of individuals from those that require actions at community and national level. Furthermore, fighting poverty, challenging injustice and working for political change are all 'behaviours' themselves. We need to understand the motivations that influence politicians to adopt policies and individuals to come together for community action and social change.

This chapter will look at the following questions:

1. What are behaviours and how can we describe them?
2. What influences human behaviour?
3. What is the role of culture, social change and economic factors in determining behaviours?
4. How do we use an understanding of behaviour, and plan health education and health promotion programmes?

Empathy – understanding other people's perspectives

We often complain because the community ignores our advice to follow healthy behaviours. Precautions to maintain health that make sense to us, are rejected by the community.

One reason for this is that we look at actions from our own point of view as health workers and place too much emphasis on health and medical factors as a reason for action. The community may consider other values to be more important, such as economic survival, status, prestige, physical beauty, attractiveness to the opposite sex, conforming to moral or religious rules and family honour. Our own motives, values, understandings may be very different from that of the community, especially if we come from different backgrounds. *What may seem to us irrational behaviour by the community can actually involve deliberate and rational decisions based on the community's own perceptions of their situation and needs.*

The approach I use in this book assumes that people are not irrational or irresponsible but try to do what they see to be the best for themselves and their families. A useful approach is 'value-expectancy theory' which suggests that people will only perform a given behaviour if *they themselves* see that it will provide some benefits, e.g. if they see breastfeeding brings about mostly good outcomes they will wish to breastfeed. If they see breastfeeding brings about mostly bad outcomes they will not wish to breastfeed.

It is *the person's own judgement* of what is a good or bad outcome that matters. What is important to us may not be considered a worthwhile outcome by the community. What is important to the community may not be important to us – but we must still respect it. It is our task as health educators to ensure that the community's judgement is based on a sound understanding of the consequences of alternative actions.

A good example of the importance of understanding the community's perspective comes from experiences in family planning programmes such as in India. Planners and health educators put effort into family planning because they were worried that the growing population was using up available resources. In their educational messages they emphasized national priorities and the cost of food, clothing and school fees. These issues were important to the planners and health educators who usually came from urban middle-class backgrounds. However, as shown in Figure 2.1, the community viewed it differently. For poor people, having more children made good sense: extra children were more hands to help in the home and fields as well as sources of care and support in their old age. They also knew from experience that some of their children would probably die of childhood diseases so they needed to have extra children to make certain enough survived. As a result of evaluating these early experiences, many in India now feel that family planning programmes will only succeed if they are part of a general health programme and accompanied by measures attacking poverty.

Planner's

If you have fewer children you will be able to spend more money on each and have a higher standard of living

You will have fewer mouths to feed

The country cannot produce enough food for everyone, build sufficient schools, provide health services and jobs

Individual's

More children will mean more help in the home and fields

We can send some to the city to work

Enough will survive to look after me in my old age

Fig. 2.1 Different perspectives on family planning

To understand why people do or do not perform a particular behaviour we have to try to find out how the community – e.g. the pregnant woman, child, elderly person, village elder – *themselves* look at the action.

Imagine you are a villager. Consider one of the behaviours mentioned in the previous chapters such as breastfeeding, building a latrine, bringing a child for measles immunization and coming for ante-natal care. Write down what you think might appear to the villager the benefits of performing the behaviour and compare them with what they might see as disadvantages. Now imagine you are a health worker trying to promote the behaviour in the community. Are there any differences between the health worker and the community in the way they see advantages and disadvantages?

This process of putting ourselves in the other person's position is called empathy. People who have lived in cities or who have gone for further education, can find it difficult to understand how rural people think and feel. Chapter 4 will give examples of how it is possible to use exercises such as role-plays to help ourselves understand the difference between the community's feelings and values and our own.

Defining the behaviour

A starting-point for understanding the factors that influence people's decisions about adopting a behaviour is to define the behaviour in as much detail as possible. This involves specifying not only *what* the behaviour is but *who* is to carry it out and *when*.

It is difficult to analyse vaguely-stated behaviours such as 'sanitation' – but easier with more precise statements which specify the type of latrine and required building materials. Terms such as 'hygiene practices' and 'family planning' apply to *groups* of behaviours. Family planning can include vasectomy, female sterilization and the contraceptive pill. Hygiene includes washing of hands with soap, food preparation, clean storage of drinking water, disposal of infants' faeces. Each of these behaviours is influenced by different factors.

By specifying the behaviours in detail, we can begin to consider some of the difficulties families face in putting our advice into practice. It is not enough just to speak of growth monitoring, immunization, weaning and child spacing. By defining immunization and growth monitoring in terms of a person bringing the child to a clinic it becomes obvious that you need to find out how accessible these services are and if mothers/caretakers have the time to bring the child. For weaning it is important to be clear what foods should be given, how frequently and when, and of the need for continuing breastfeeding for as long as possible.

A good example of the importance of specifying the behaviour at the beginning of a programme is the use of oral rehydration solution (ORS) for children with diarrhoea. You will have to decide whether it is appropriate in that particular community to promote the use of packets or home-made solution. If you choose home-made, you will have to decide whether to base it on salt/sugar, rice/other cereal solutions or readily available home fluids. You will also have to consider the type of containers to make up the solution, how much ORS to give and when to start giving it to the child. The World Health Organization now recommends that diarrhoea should be first treated in the home with any available fluid including water (some local 'bush' teas might not be suitable). ORS should only be used if there are signs of dehydration. Only when you have made these decisions on the type of ORS can you begin to analyze possible obstacles to adoption of ORS in your community and decide what to include in your educational programme.

You can begin to make judgements about the feasibility of changing a behaviour once you have described it carefully and considered the following questions:

How often should it be performed – daily, every few days, occasionally, only once?
How complicated is it to carry out – is it very simple or does it require learning new skills?
How similar is it to existing practices – is it completely new, or does it show some similarities?
How easily does it fit in with existing practices – is it totally incompatible, partly compatible or does it fit in with existing practices?
How much does it cost, in time, money or resources to carry out the behaviour?
Does the behaviour fit in with a felt need of the community?
How much impact will the behaviour have on health – a great deal, very little?
Will beneficial effects be observed in the short or long term – within a few weeks, months or years?

You can predict a great deal from the answers to these questions. Hygiene behaviours such as cleaning children and washing hands have to be done every day. They will be more difficult to promote than a behaviour such as immunization that only has to be done a few times. Behaviours which involve spending time or money, require learning new skills or conflict with existing practices will be more difficult to promote than ones that are simple to carry out and fit in with existing practices. *Customs* and *traditions* are behaviours that have been carried out for a long time and have been handed down from parents to children. They will be more difficult to change than behaviours that have been recently acquired and held only by individuals.

Sometimes our analysis of the influences on a behaviour will tell us that it is not realistic to attempt to promote a particular behaviour because of the enabling factors that would be required. A good example of this is the boiling of drinking water. Boiling of drinking water requires time for supervision and for the water to cool. Fuel is required which must be paid for or collected. A family must have a suitable cooking pot and an appropriate storage container for the water.

You will have more impact if you advise behaviours appropriate to people's income and culture. For example, if people do not eat particular foods, you can develop nutrition advice that does not involve those foods. As a general rule you should make your advice fit the community rather than expect them to change to suit you.

Behavioural intention and enabling factors

You should try to avoid putting the blame for a failure of a health education programme on lack of interest or motivation on the part of the community. The distinguished health educator Lawrence Green developed a useful concept that he called *enabling factors*. Sometimes a person may intend to perform a behaviour but still not do so. This is because of the influence of enabling factors such as time, money, equipment, skills or health services.

Enabling factors for a mother to give oral rehydration solution to her child with diarrhoea would be: time, containers, salt and sugar and knowledge of how to prepare and administer it. Enabling factors for a latrine programme would be: money, essential components, e.g. slabs and the necessary construction skills. For behavioural intention——► behaviour change

enabling factors

time
money and material resources
special skills required
appropriate and accessible health services

Fig. 2.2 Enabling factors

a family planning programme, enabling factors would be availability of contraceptives, accessible family planning services and the necessary skills for using the particular method. Convenient and accessible services are important enabling factors for the utilization of child health services or antenatal clinics.

You should ensure that when the public make the effort to follow your health education advice that the required services such as screening facilities, medicines, vaccines, building materials, etc. are actually available.

Money can be another important enabling factor! Many health education programmes have failed because they did not consider the poverty and social inequalities that often underlie a particular behaviour. Social inequalities present a serious challenge to the improvement of health.

A neglected enabling factor is the *time* to carry out the health-promoting actions. Most of the important child care practices promoted in the 'Facts for Life' programme described in the previous chapter will require additional time caring for the child, taking the child to clinics, giving ORS, etc. In most situations it is the mother who is expected to undertake these extra tasks. However, women in developing (and developed) countries are already overworked with *multiple roles* that include looking after the home, fetching water and fuel, caring for children, taking children to the child health clinic, preparing meals, growing food and going out to work. Their workload increases in particular seasons such as planting and harvesting when there is more agricultural work. These busy times of the year often coincide with seasonal peaks in food shortages and diseases such as diarrhoea. It is unrealistic to expect women to take action to improve health and nutrition unless we find ways of reducing their workload to give them time to follow our advice.

Social pressure

One reason health education programmes fail is that they are directed at individuals and ignore the influences of other people. Few people make decisions or perform actions without considering the opinions and views of those around them.

Fig. 2.3 A woman's work is never done

Think about your own family and friends. Whom do you consult when you have to make an important decision? As you can see in Figure 2.4, we are all influenced by the various persons in our *social network*. Some people may want you to take action – others may oppose you. Exactly who has the most influence will depend both on the particular individual and the culture of the community. For example, in some societies the mother-in-law is particularly influential; in others, it may be the elders, including uncles.

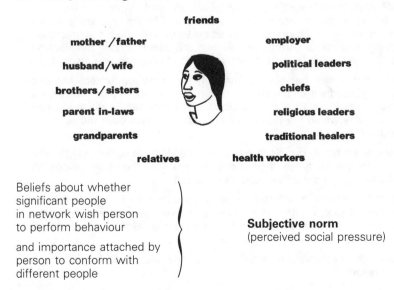

Fig. 2.4 The influence of social pressure

The influential people – called *significant others* – change during a person's life. In a young child it is usually the parents who have the most influence. As a child grows older, friends become important and a young person can feel a powerful pressure to conform to the 'peer group'. Examples of the importance of social pressure are: the woman who does not adopt family planning because her husband disapproves; the young man who starts smoking because his friends encourage him to do so; the mother who wants to give oral rehydration solution to the child but the grandmother objects; the child who cleans his teeth because his mother insists; and the family who built a latrine because the religious leader in the community wanted them to do so.

Pressure from others can be a positive influence to adopt health-promoting practices as well as an obstacle. In real life we are constantly under pressure to act in different ways. Some people may approve of us doing something, others may be against. How we respond will depend on whose opinions have the most influence on us. For example, a woman may believe that her friends and the health worker wish her to build a latrine but her father and husband do not. She is likely to conform to the wishes of those most important to her. The term 'subjective norm' was introduced by the psychologist Fishbein to describe the overall perceived social pressure.

I have listed some questions that you can ask to find out the influences of social pressure in your community.

Questions to ask to find out about social pressures

Who are the most influential people in the community? Are there informal leaders who are looked to for decisions although they remain in the background? What qualities tend to make people's opinion carry weight in the community (money, children, age, education, cattle, wives)?

In what areas of life, e.g. economic, child care, food production, do the various leaders have influence? What leaders within the community are most likely to make decisions that influence community health, the delivery of health care in the area, or various aspects of the health programme? What do they think about the practices that you are trying to promote? Are there differences of views among the leaders? Could local leaders be involved in your health education? How can you reach them?

How important is family membership in community life? How are families and kinship groups typically organized within the culture? What roles do the father, mother, son, daughter, grandparents (or other persons typically part of the family within a certain culture) commonly play within the family? Where and how does each member typically spend his time?

How and by whom are family decisions typically made? Who is consulted? What is the typical timing for various types of decisions? Where does the power within the family appear to lie? How do they feel about outsiders?

Who generally makes various health-related decisions within the family (i.e. what to do when a member is sick, whether to take certain preventive measures, what the family will eat, what money can be allotted for health-related expenses, whether a sick member may follow certain medical advice)?

Do children ever make health-related decisions? Are they taken seriously if their views differ from their parents?

Fig. 2.5 An Oba (traditional chief) from Nigeria – an example of traditional authority

Culture and behaviour

Most people agree that culture has an important influence on behaviour. It is common to hear the terms cultural practice, cultural belief, cultural value and cultural norm. However, culture is a misunderstood term and actually consists of three overlapping features: shared characteristics, traditions and belief systems.

Shared characteristics

A behaviour, value or belief can be shared by a group of people, a whole community or even a country. The term sub-culture can also be applied to a group such as teenagers, soldiers, factory workers when we consider their special characteristics. Other words for shared characteristics are *norms or customs* – i.e. something that is common or normal for that group.

Traditions

These are practices that have been maintained for a long time and passed down from parents to children. Another word for this process of handing down from one generation to another is socialization. 'Primary socialization' is the term for the learning that takes place from one's family during the first five years. During this period language, habits, values, beliefs and rules of behaviour are learnt. This happens by the child following the instructions of the parent as well as the more informal process of copying the actions of adults.

Belief systems

While some behaviours exist on their own, others are part of a wider system of beliefs such as religion or a traditional medicine system. For example, in one person avoidance of pork may be simply a matter of not liking the taste. In another person that behaviour might be because the person is a Jew or Muslim.

31

A great deal is learnt during
early years from the family
– this process is called
primary socialization.

Many characteristics are
shared by different people
in a community – norms.

Fig. 2.6 Traditions and norms

We can apply these three components of culture – shared characteristics, traditions and a system of beliefs, to the processes listed here which all influence health and health education activities.

Different ways in which culture can influence health

life-cycle: family structure, patterns of influence among family members, role of women, children, rituals and roles surrounding birth, growing up, relations with other people, sex and marriage; family formation, work, growing old, death;
patterns of living and consumption: clothing; housing; child rearing, food production, storage and consumption; hygiene practices; sanitation;
health and illness behaviours: concepts of health and illness; ideas about mental illness and handicap; care of sick people; traditional medicine systems; patterns of help-seeking when ill; use of doctors and traditional healers; concepts about the biological workings of the body, growth, conception, pregnancy, birth etc.;
patterns of communication: language; verbal and non-verbal communication; taboos on public discussion of sensitive items; vocabulary of the language; oral traditions;
religion and 'world view': ideas about the meaning of life and death; rituals surrounding important life events; ideals about the possibility and desirability of change;
patterns of social and political organization: political structures; community leadership and authority; divisions and social inequalities;
economic patterns/types of employment: ideas about wealth and income; ownership of land; use of money and barter; savings and credit arrangements.

'A state of complete physical, mental and social well-being, not merely the absence of disease or infirmity.' WHO (1946)

'The nearest approach to health is a physical and mental state fairly free of discomfort and pain, which permits the person concerned to function as effectively and as long as possible in the environment where chance or choice has placed him.' Dubos

'The Yoruba generic concept for health is *Alafia*. In its literal sense *Alafia* means peace. The word embraces the totality of an individual's physical, social, emotional, psychological and spiritual well-being in the total environmental setting. The Yorubas believe that the possession of *Alafia* is a result of the dynamic interaction of all those variables. According to the people: *"Eni ba l'Alafia l'ohun gbogbo"* (Whoever has health has all things) and *"Alafia l'ogun oso"* (Health is wealth).' Ademuwagun (1978) Nigeria

According to Indian philosophy, the universe consists of five gross elements – earth, water, fire, air and the ethereal parts of the sky – and the same factors constitute the basic elements of the human body. However, in a human body, life does not depend only on these five bodily components but also on the presence of normally functioning sense organs and of the mind and soul. Thus Sushruta defined the healthy person as follows: "He is the healthy man who possesses the balance of body hormones, proper functioning of all the body elements and who has the pleasant disposition of mind, soul and sense organs." ' Valupa (1975)

Health – an ancient concept rooted in culture

Health itself is a concept determined by culture and society and we may each have our own ideas about what it means to be healthy. Health is so important to basic functions of survival that it is not very surprising that most societies in the world have well-established ideas about health.

In looking at these definitions of health some significant points emerge. Despite the broad nature of the WHO definition, many doctors and health workers still see health in terms of diseases and disease prevention. However, traditional ideas of health in Asian, African and European cultures have a wider *holistic* view. Health can be:

- a feeling of well-being;
- the opportunity of achieving fulfilling activities;
- a balance of physical and mental states;
- achievement of one's potential; or
- ability to cope with life's demands.

Many different traditional medicine systems are practised throughout the world. Traditional healers may be widely respected and are consulted by a wide range of people. In the past they were criticized and called 'quacks' and 'witch doctors'. It is now realized that they have an important role to play and that efforts should be directed towards integrating them within primary health care. Some of the questions you will need to find out in your community about health systems are listed here.

Concepts of health and illness: What do people in the community generally consider a state of good health or illness/poor health consists of? What conditions of the body are considered normal and abnormal? What is considered to be a physical 'handicap'? What are their feelings towards people who have abnormalities or are disabled? What priority does the value of 'good health' have within the community? How important is health compared to other needs and values?

Coping with illness: What types of actions do families take when a member becomes ill or injured? Are particular family or community members involved in the prevention, diagnosis or treatment of certain illnesses of other family members? Are there special family medicines, remedies, treatments? Do family health beliefs and practices differ from your health education messages?

What are the typical attitudes within a culture toward the sick? Who decides within a culture if a person is ill? How is the sick person expected to behave? Does the person consult family or traditional healers first before consulting Western practitioners? What methods do traditional healers use?

Beliefs about health, disease, treatment and prevention: What general beliefs do various community people have concerning cause, prevention, diagnosis and treatment of diseases in general or of specific ones? Are there any particular methods people use to help maintain their own health or that of others? Are there any special traditional theories of disease to which certain people adhere? Do they still believe them? What is the general understanding of and attitude towards Western medical explanations and practices?

What are the attitudes of persons of various ages, sexes, ethnic groups and religions towards the body? Towards discussing the body? Towards self-examination? What beliefs do people have concerning the organs and systems of the body and how they function?

General beliefs concerning health and illness behaviours: What are people's beliefs concerning immunizations, various screening tests, preventive health measures, hygiene, prevention of accidents and other behaviours you may be trying to promote in the community? Are there any special beliefs, rules, preferences or prejudices concerning foods? Are foods used to treat diseases? What do the people feel should be an ideal diet? Does this change at different ages and special states, e.g. in pregnancy?

How is knowledge concerning sex acquired by growing children? What are the social and cultural beliefs and practices surrounding sexual intercourse (premarital intercourse, contacting sex partners, homosexuality, bisexuality, techniques of sexual intercourse, sexual restrictions, extramarital intercourse)?

There are many different kinds of traditional medicine. Some of these, including the Hindu Ayurvedic medicine, the Chinese Yin/Yang system and homeopathic medicine are complex medical 'systems' with written books, training colleges and registration procedures for recognition. Others are small-scale, informal and passed on through oral traditions and healers taking on 'apprentices' to study under them. The anthropologist George Foster suggests that traditional medical systems can be grouped into the two categories in Table 2.1. The first group, 'personalistic', includes systems of medicine where the blame for illness is put on supernatural forces, witchcraft, spirits or the 'evil eye'. In the second group, are 'naturalistic' reasons for illness based on 'natural' explanations including theories of the body, actions of herbs, etc.

Fig. 2.7 Traditional healers: (left) China and (right) Zambia

Table 2.1 Types of traditional medical systems

	Supernatural	'Natural' explanations
Illness explained by	Active purposeful intervention of another person or supernatural agent, e.g. through witchcraft, evil eye, spirits.	Explanations not based on supernatural influences but in terms of concepts of health and disease – e.g. lack of balance of factors in body, hot/cold theories, yin/yang, etc.
Extent to which same explanation for illness also applies for other misfortunes	Illness is only a special case of wider misfortune.	Explanations limited to disease only, not other disasters or misfortunes.
Levels of causation	Thinking about causes on different levels – not just cause of illness but who has caused it.	Single level of cause – do not ask questions such as who caused the disease.
Diagnosis	Powerful witch doctors or spiritualists needed to identify who has caused the illness. Treatment less important.	Patient seeks aid for curers for relief of symptoms and not to find out what has happened.
Nature of curers	Curers are needed who have supernatural or magical divining power.	Curers tend to be 'doctors' in that they have learnt their skills through observation and practice and not through divine intervention.

Values

Values are characteristics held to be important and prized by an individual or community. Usually values are qualities at an abstract level such as bravery and intelligence. A person's values might be reflected in the way he or she completes the following statement: '*The things that are important to me are . . . .*' Examples of characteristics that can be valued by communities include:

being a good mother	having many children
being approved by friends	owning a large number of cattle
having the respect of my community	being strong
being attractive to the opposite sex	masculinity and sexual prowess
being 'modern'	having many children
being healthy	

A person may have his or her own individual values. However, values are usually part of culture and shared at a community or national level. Health is only one of many possible values and a person may feel that other values such as fame, wealth or respect in the community may be more important.

We can sometimes bring about changes by emphasizing values which do not involve health. For example, we might explain to a woman that breastfeeding her child will bring her weight down after delivery and make her look more attractive. We might persuade a person to build a latrine by emphasizing the benefits of privacy or of being considered modern by one's neighbours.

In health education we are often trying to promote health as a value or encourage people to think about their values. This process is called *value-clarification* and is usually carried out through small group discussion.

It is important to take care to avoid imposing your own values on the community – base your messages on what people *themselves* feel to be important.

Beliefs

Beliefs deal with a people's understanding of themselves and their environment. Beliefs about the different possible outcomes from performing actions are especially important in understanding behaviour. I list some types of beliefs that are important in health education as well as examples of each.

Fig. 2.8 Planners and facilitators must strive to understand the beliefs that influence behaviour...(SEARO cartoon)

Causes of diseases	*Lung cancer is caused by smoking.*
	Accidents are caused by sorcery.
How easily prevented a disease is	*Using a pit latrine will prevent hookworm.*
	Immunization will prevent measles.
	Methods of prevention of having children do not exist.
Effort involved in taking action	*Building a pit latrine costs a lot of money.*
	The health centre is very far away.
Benefits resulting from taking action	*Taking part in a primary health care programme will improve our village.*
Consequences of disease	*Measles does not lead to death.*
	Diarrhoea causes death.
Personal susceptibility to 'disease'	*My children will not catch measles.*
	I am not likely to get pregnant again.
What is normal or a state of disease	*Malaria is very common here.*
	Most people have six children.
	Diarrhoea is a normal state of growing up.
What other persons think you should do	*My husband would disapprove of my using family planning.*
Beliefs about the possibility of change	*There is nothing I can do to grow more food.*
	Having children is the will of God and I cannot change it.
Credibility of communication source	*The nurse does not care about my baby.*
	Our village level worker knows very little.
Beliefs about prestige/status	*Bottle feeding is practised by modern women.*
	Building a pit latrine will make people look up to me.

How beliefs are formed

It is important to find out how a particular belief has been acquired in order to predict how easily it might be changed. A belief might have been formed from an individual or community's personal experiences, e.g. they may have visited a latrine and found it smelly; tried a folk remedy and felt better afterwards; attended a clinic and found long queues; seen a child receive an immunization and then get measles (e.g. through poorly-kept vaccines), etc. It is difficult to change those beliefs which have arisen through a person's direct experience unless you can provide a practical demonstration.

The study of medical anthropology provides valuable insights into how particular beliefs can be part of wider belief systems such as religions and traditional medical systems. If a belief is part of a wider system of beliefs it can be very difficult to change, e.g. a pregnant woman in the Indian sub-continent might hold the belief that she should not eat eggs, as part of a general concept of hot/cold states of the body and foods.

A person also develops beliefs from what he/she reads or hears from other persons. For example, many beliefs are acquired during childhood from our parents and others in our family or community through *primary socialization*. At

Fig. 2.9 Our beliefs have many origins – which do you think might be more difficult to change?

each stage of the human life cycle from pre-school, school, young adult upwards, beliefs can be formed. It can be difficult to change those beliefs which have been held since childhood or have been acquired from trusted persons in the community.

The Health Belief Model

The Health Belief Model (HBM) was developed by Rosenstock and Becker to explain why people did not use health services (utilization behaviour), but has been applied to many aspects of health behaviour as well. According to the HBM, if a person is to perform a particular act such as go for screening for cancer, he/she has to:

believe they are *susceptible*	that the health problem could affect him or her personally – rather than other people or society as a whole.
feel that it was *serious*	that the health problem could lead to death or other serious outcomes if action was not taken.
believe it could be *prevented*	that taking the action would prevent the health problem and that the benefits of taking action would outweigh the disadvantages.

A man may accept alcoholism as serious and that it can be prevented but may not believe that *he* was susceptible and could become an alcoholic. Then you should not waste effort emphasizing the seriousness of alcoholism but concentrate on making him realize that he could be at risk. A woman may believe that her child could get measles and that this would have serious consequences. However, she may not believe that measles can be prevented by immunization. In that case you should base your communications strategy on the message that immunization prevents measles.

The Health Belief Model provides a useful checklist for choosing the points to emphasize in any communication message – especially the importance of perceived seriousness, susceptibility and preventability. But it has some weaknesses: it does not consider social pressure from others in the family or community and ignores enabling factors. These are both taken into account in the BASNEF Model described in the next section.

Attitudes and Fishbein

Attitudes and beliefs are frequently confused. The psychologist Fishbein suggested that the term attitude should be used for a person's judgement of a behaviour as good or bad and worth carrying out. This judgement will depend on the beliefs held about the consequences of performing the behaviour. A person will normally hold a range of beliefs about the possible good and bad consequences of performing a particular behaviour. For example, a mother may believe that breastfeeding will improve the health of her baby but may also believe that it will make her appear old-fashioned. If, overall, a person believes that performing the behaviour will lead to mainly good outcomes, then the attitude will be favourable. If the outcomes are perceived as mainly bad, the attitude to the behaviour will be unfavourable.

Whether the overall judgement (i.e. attitude) of the behaviour is favourable or unfavourable will also depend on the values placed on the different possible consequences e.g. in the latrine example, the values placed on health, privacy, owning a bicycle, foul smells, flies, appearing progressive, etc. A particular consequence may be perceived as a bad one by one person, but acceptable (and even an advantage!) by another.

According to Fishbein, whether or not a person forms an intention to perform a behaviour will also depend on the overall pressure from those around him, i.e. *subjective norm*. A person may judge the proposed behaviour favourably but may

My building a pit latrine will result in:
being seen to be progressive
not being able to afford a bicycle
improving the health of my family
greater privacy than going to the bush
foul smells close to the house
nuisance from flies
gaining approval from the chief.

beliefs about different
possible consequences
that person perceives might
arise from performing behaviour

extent to which each consequence
is seen to be good or bad

overall **ATTITUDE**
(judgement) towards
behaviour as good
or bad

Fig. 2.10   Role of beliefs in forming attitude

perceive that those important to him do not want him to perform the behaviour. A person may not have a favourable attitude towards the behaviour but be pressurized by those around him to perform it. Whether or not the person's own judgement can overcome the influence of those around him will depend on the individual's strength of will and susceptibility to pressure. There can be considerable cultural pressure on individuals to conform to family and community influence. Fishbein's model is a significant improvement on the Health Belief Model because it considers both an individual's beliefs and the social pressures from others in the family and community.

Putting it all together – BASNEF

I have put together the BASNEF model (the name comes from the first letters of Beliefs, Attitude, Subjective Norm and Enabling Factor) by combining the approach by Fishbein discussed in the previous section and the concept of enabling factors introduced by Lawrence Green; it is summarized in Figure 2.11. It should be seen as a checklist for programme planning rather than a complete description of the complex processes that underlie a person's actions.

Using BASNEF to plan health education and health promotion

Applying the BASNEF approach involves examining behaviour from the perspective of the community. This is not as easy as it sounds as, even if you share their background, your education and health training will make you look at issues differently. You will need to speak to individuals and groups at the beginning of

Fig. 2.11 Summary of BASNEF model for understanding behaviour

enabling factors   beliefs/attitudes   subjective norms

Fig. 2.12 Three possible reactions to a talk

a health education session to find out about the underlying factors, including beliefs, values, social pressure and enabling factors that influence the community. You can use the questions in the lists on social influence, health beliefs and beliefs in this chapter to form the basis for choosing what questions to answer. If resources are available, you can carry out this questioning more systematically as an organized survey or 'community diagnosis'.

Once sufficient background information is available on the various factors in the BASNEF model, making decisions on health education and health promotion approaches involves the following steps.

41

1. **Make sure the behaviour will improve health.** Before devoting time and energy to promoting a behaviour, make sure that it will actually benefit the community. It is still common to find health educators wasting effort trying to persuade people to give up harmless behaviours or take up new behaviours for which there is little evidence of health benefits.

2. **Make sure the behaviour change you are asking for is a realistic one.** Avoid behaviours that are complicated, require enabling factors such as time, money or new skills and do not fit in with the culture and present practices.

   Can the proposed behaviour be changed to make it more acceptable, cheaper and easier to carry out? You might be able to reduce the cost by developing low-cost solutions such as cheaper latrines, heat-efficient ovens, etc. An *appropriate technology* should be compatible with the culture of the community, technically feasible using locally-available skills and materials, require minimum maintenance and be simple to use. For example, in the case of sanitation, if your analysis of culture and beliefs indicates that the community prefer sitting to squatting, you should design latrines with seats. If it is acceptable to build latrines in a spiral shape without doors you can avoid the cost of doors.

3. **Provide necessary enabling factors.** Your communication programme should make sure that the required enabling factors are available. This could involve setting up community organization programmes aimed at improving living conditions such as income, housing, water supply, agriculture and sanitation. It may be necessary to improve the situation of women to provide the additional time required to carry out the behaviour. Health services can be reorganized to make them accessible and more appropriate services, e.g. mobile clinics and home visits, introduced where necessary. You can include opportunities for the community to learn any special skills needed to put the advice into practice.

   You can find out whether enabling factors are needed by careful questioning. A good example of this is the question that the nutritionist Judith Brown asks first when planning a nutrition intervention. *'Does the family have sufficient resources to grow or buy the necessary food?'*

   If NO Then tackle the food availability issue first and find ways of improving their economic position so that they can obtain the food.
   If YES Then explore other reasons why they may not prepare the food such as lack of time, necessary knowledge or beliefs.

   Tackling enabling factors can involve moving well beyond the traditional range of activities for health services. This often involves *intersectoral collaboration* – working with field personnel from other services such as agriculture, rural development, adult education and cooperatives. You may have to challenge vested interests at the local level and become involved in action at a national level to influence government policies.

4. **Consider social pressures from the family and community.** If the enabling factors are all readily available, then the barrier to change may be social pressure on the person – the subjective norm. It is unreasonable to expect a person, no matter how convinced, to go against the wishes of those around him or her in the community. Giving advice to the individual at the clinic would not be enough. You must go into the community and convince the influential 'opinion leaders' in the family and community. For example, you could set up demonstration latrines at their homes. You could look for opinion leaders who have successfully changed their lifestyle and would be happy to talk

to others and explain the benefits of giving up smoking, using oral rehydration therapy, using a latrine, adopting child spacing, etc. People are often more easily persuaded by people they trust and believe. These 'satisfied acceptors' can be a powerful help in your educational programmes.

5. **Identify any beliefs that might influence the person's attitude.** The issue of changing the beliefs that influence a person's attitude has deliberately been left until last. This is because the blame for failure has often been put on 'bad beliefs' and 'laziness' and health education programmes often fail to take into account the enabling factors and social pressure described above.

If the community believes that performing the behaviour will lead to unfavourable outcomes you should try to find out why. You might be able to change the proposed behaviour to make it more acceptable. If this is not possible – and there is clear evidence of health benefits from changing the behaviour – then it is justifiable to try to change beliefs. You could try to strengthen those beliefs which link performing the behaviour to outcomes that the community considers desirable.

Earlier in this chapter I discussed the origins of beliefs and showed how you can predict which beliefs are the easiest to change. If it is just the individual who holds a particular belief then it might be possible to influence the belief by discussions only with that person. More often, however, the belief is also held by others in the community as part of their shared culture. It is then necessary to direct effort at groups of people rather than individuals.

The community is more likely to be convinced if the benefits of a behaviour can clearly be shown in an observable demonstration, e.g. that a well-designed latrine does not smell, immunization is effective, oral rehydration therapy prevents death. It is usually easier to influence those beliefs that have only been acquired recently, are held by individuals and not by the whole community, come from sources that are not highly respected and are not part of a religion or traditional medical system.

6. **Find out whether the influences on behaviour operate at the individual, family, community or higher level.** Health education can be criticized for over-emphasizing working with individuals and failing to work at other levels such as the family, community, national and international levels where many influences on behaviour operate (see Figure 1.8).

Many of the problems of selection of unrealistic and inappropriate messages and behaviour changes can be resolved by working at the community level and building in community participation in the selection of objectives. Working at this level can create opportunities to *empower* communities to tackle problems. If it is necessary that traditional practices must change, then it is important that the community makes the decisions as to how these changes should take place.

Poor health may be because of problems at a community level or national decisions. Other influences at the national level are agricultural policies or commercial advertising. You may have to try to influence governments to adopt health-promoting policies such as the restriction of health-damaging activities like the advertising of baby milk and tobacco. The use of non-formal education techniques to generate community participation, raise consciousness and stimulate action on social and economic determinants of health will be described further in the chapters on 'Working with communities' and 'Politics and health'.

Influences		Actions needed
culture values traditions mass media education experiences	**BELIEFS ATTITUDES**	Communication programmes to modify beliefs and values directed at individual or whole community
health services income/poverty women's status inequalities employment agriculture transport	**ENABLING FACTORS**	Programmes to improve health services, situation of women, income, agriculture, housing, water supply, skill training
family community social network culture social change power structures family structure	**SUBJECTIVE NORM** (social pressure)	Communication *directed* at persons in family and community who have influence

Fig. 2.13 Influences on behaviour and choice of communication strategies

Summary

This chapter has reviewed influences on human behaviour and has introduced an approach I have called BASNEF. The starting point for our analysis has been the individual person's behaviour. However, an understanding of the influences on behaviour can lead to interventions that go beyond the individual to include programmes at the family, community and national levels and involve both educational, social, economic and political change.

1. Have you drawn upon available current knowledge to make sure that the behaviours chosen will have an impact on prevention?
2. Can you choose behaviours that are:
   - simple to carry out and require few additional skills or resources?
   - compatible with local culture and acceptable to the community?
   - meet a felt need in the community and are wanted?
   - produce some benefits in the short term that are observable?
3. Are enabling factors such as money, time and materials required for performing the behaviour? If so, how can we make sure that they are provided?
4. If your programmes involve mother and child health, have you taken into account the workload of women in the home and fields?
5. Who are the significant persons in the family or community who have influence over the particular behaviour? Do they support your programme?
6. What beliefs does the community have about the consequences of performing the behaviour? How were these beliefs formed? Can the unfavourable perceptions be reduced? Can the positive beliefs be strengthened?
7. Should you direct your efforts at the individual, family, district, national or international level? How can you encourage community participation in the understanding of behaviour and planning of health education programmes? What changes in government policy are needed to make healthy choices easier?

3. An introduction to communication

Communication involves the transfer between people of information including ideas, emotions, knowledge and skills. This chapter will:

1. Explore the psychological and social processes involved in communication, reasons for communication failure and provide guidelines for successful communication.
2. Examine the relative influences of source, message, channel and receiver on the communication process and consider how this understanding can help in designing communication programmes.
3. Consider how an understanding of pictures and visual perception can help in designing visual communications and audio-visual aids.
4. Explore the main characteristics of a range of communication methods – in particular face-to-face and mass media.
5. Provide a theoretical basis for later chapters in this book that look at the role of communication in teaching, mass media, community participation, working with people and use of folk media.

Fig. 3.1 Human communication

Table 3.1 Examples of failure at different communication stages

	Immunization poster	Water/sanitation	Radio nutrition	How to ensure success
Reaches SENSES; is seen or heard	Poster is placed at the health centre and only seen by mothers who have already immunized their children.	Only men, not women, were at the public meeting. The women did not hear about water programme.	The radio programme was broadcast at a time when the women were working in the fields.	*Research target group to find out where they go, what are their listening, viewing, reading habits.*
Gains ATTENTION; holds interest, is noticed	The poster lacks striking features and does not stand out compared with attractive commercial advertisements.	The sanitation exhibition at the agricultural show was boring so most people walked past.	The nutrition programme was boring, so the women switched to the other station.	*Find out interests of target group. Make programme interesting, attractive, and unusual. Test it out.*
is UNDERSTOOD; correctly interpreted	Poster showing large hypodermic syringe held by smiling doctor was thought by the community to be a devil with a knife.	The field worker used complicated words such as faecal-borne diseases, stools and bacteria. No one understood.	The women were confused by the technical terms, vitamins, proteins and xeropthalmia.	*Make it simple, avoid confusing language. Pre-test words and pictures with sample of intended target group.*
is ACCEPTED, believed; learning takes place	People believe that measles is caused by witchcraft and do not believe the poster even though they understand the message.	The fieldworker explained that diseases were passed by bacteria and faeces. The people laughed at this explanation.	The announcer was a young girl and the women did not believe that she could know anything about children.	*Base message on what people already believe. Use credible sources. Pre-test messages for acceptability.*
CHANGES BEHAVIOUR	The mother accepted the message and wished to take child for immunization but the grandmother did not allow it.	They were convinced of the importance of pit latrines and wanted to build them. But they did not have any cement for slabs.	The women wanted to put the advice into practice but did not have money to buy the food.	*Target the influential people and ensure enabling factors are available. Pre-test for feasibility.*
IMPROVES HEALTH	The vaccine was destroyed by a break in the cold chain and the child became sick with measles.	They followed the advice and built latrines. But the children were afraid to use them so the levels of diarrhoea did not reduce.	The women followed the advice and bought their children expensive protein foods – but stopped breastfeeding. The children developed malnutrition.	*Choose most important behaviours. Make sure support services are functioning.*

Communication stages

Communication can involve ordinary conversation, such as explaining a point, asking a question or just talking to pass the time. However, in health education and health promotion we communicate for a special purpose – to promote improvements in health through the modification of the human, social and political factors that influence behaviours. To achieve these objectives, a successful communication must pass through several stages (Figure 3.2) – and, at each stage, communication failure can take place (see Table 3.1).

Fig. 3.2 Communication stages

Stage 1: reaching the intended audience

Communication cannot be effective unless it is seen or heard by its intended audience. This may seem obvious and does not require any complex theories to explain. But many programmes fail even at this simple stage. A common cause of failure is *preaching to the converted*, e.g. posters placed at the clinic or talks given at the antenatal clinics. These only reach the people who attend the services and are already motivated.

But the groups you are trying to reach may not attend clinics, nor have radios or newspapers. They may be busy working at the time when the health education programmes are broadcast. Communications should be directed where people are going to see them or hear them. This requires studying your intended audience to find out where they might see posters, what their listening and reading habits are.

Stage 2: attracting the audience's attention

Any communication must attract attention so that people will make the effort to listen/read it. Examples of communication failures at this stage are:

- walking past the poster without bothering to look at it;
- not paying attention to the health talk or demonstration at the clinic;
- not stopping at the exhibition at the showground; and
- turning off the radio programme or switching over.

At any one time we receive a wide range of information from each of our five senses – touch, smell, vision, hearing and taste. It is impossible to concentrate on all this at the same time. Attention is the name of the process by which a person selects part of this complex mixture to focus on (i.e. *to pay attention to*) while ignoring others for the time being. Some of the psychological processes that influence the way a message can attract an audience's attention will be discussed later in this chapter.

Stage 3: understanding the message (perception)

Once a person pays attention to a message he/she then tries to understand it. Another name for this stage is perception. *Visual perception* is the term used for understanding of visual messages and *pictorial perception* for understanding of pictures. Perception is a highly *subjective* process – two people may hear the same radio programme or see the same poster and interpret the message quite differently from each other and from the meaning intended by the sender.

A person's interpretation of a communication will depend on many things. Misunderstandings can easily take place when: complex language and unfamiliar technical words are used; pictures contain complicated diagrams and distracting details; show unfamiliar subjects; or familiar objects shown from an unusual view. Another reason for misunderstanding is when too much information is presented and people cannot absorb it all. More information on visual perception is given later in this chapter.

Stage 4: promoting change (acceptance)

A communication should not only be received and understood – it should be believed and accepted. In Chapter 2 some of the reasons why a particular belief might be difficult to change were discussed. It is easier to change beliefs when they have been acquired only recently. It is more difficult to influence a belief that has been held for a long time or if people already have well-developed beliefs on the topic (which is often the case). It is usually easier to promote a belief when its effects can be easily demonstrated, e.g. that ventilated, improved pit latrines do not smell. If a belief is held by the whole community, or is part of a wider belief system such as their religion, we can predict that it will be very difficult to change by methods such as mass media and leaflets.

Later in this chapter you will see how the nature of the source and content of the message can influence whether people believe and accept the message.

Stage 5: producing a change in behaviour

A communication may result in a change in beliefs and attitude but still not influence behaviour. This can happen when the communication has not been targeted at the belief that has the most influence on the person's attitude to the behaviour. For example, many communication programmes have emphasized the dangers of diarrhoea and failed to give enough emphasis to dehydration.

A person may have a favourable attitude and want to carry out the action, e.g. use family planning, bring the child for immunization, etc. However, pressure from other people in the family or community may prevent the person from doing it.

Another reason a person may not perform a behaviour is a lack of enabling factors such as money, time, skills or health services. The role of culture, beliefs, social pressure and enabling factors are discussed in detail in the previous chapter.

Stage 6: improvement in health

Improvements in health will only take place if the behaviours have been carefully selected so that they really do influence health. If your messages are based on outdated and incorrect ideas, people could follow your advice but their health would not improve. This need to ensure accurate advice was one reason why the

'*Facts for Life*' initiative was launched by UNICEF, WHO and UNESCO (see page 9).

Components of communications

In looking at the factors which influence the success of a communication, it is helpful to consider separately and distinguish between *receiver, source, message* and *channel*.

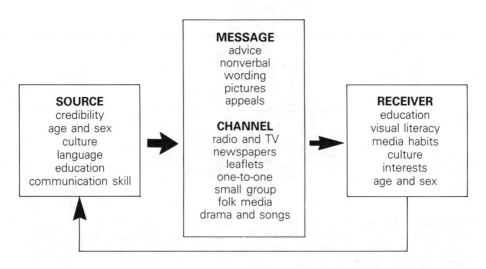

Fig. 3.3 Source, message, channel and receiver

Receiver (audience)

The first step in planning any communication is to consider the intended audience. A method that will be effective with one audience may not succeed with another. Two people may hear the same radio programme, see the same poster or attend the same talk and interpret them quite differently. Some of the main information you need to find out when planning communications are shown in Figure 3.4. You should also refer to the list of questions about patterns of influence and health beliefs on pages 30, 32 and 33.

Source

People are exposed to communications from many different sources and more likely to believe a communication from a person or organization that they trust, i.e. has high source-credibility. Think about the communities you are familiar with and ask yourself: what special qualities make a person trusted? What can make the community lose trust in a person?

In considering these questions you can refer to the discussion of opinion leaders, significant others and social pressure in the previous chapter and the detailed checklist of questions on page 30. Rural persons are not usually impressed by educational status and have more regard for personal qualities. People do not believe radio programmes or posters just because they are produced by the Ministry of Health. The health education worker is often not the most credible source. You will need to find out who your intended audience respects and involve these

Educational factors. What is their age and educational level? What kinds of arguments and appeals might convince them? Can they read? What words do they use in their everyday conversation? Are they used to looking at pictures and diagrams?
Socio-cultural factors. What do they already know, believe and feel about the topic of the communication? How strongly-held are their present beliefs? What values do they hold to be important? Whose opinions and views do they trust? How open are they to new ideas?
Pattern of communication. What patterns of communication already exist in the community? Are there any rules surrounding the discussion of health topics openly? What rules are there for conversation between people? How do people show respect when talking to another person? Where do people find out about health issues? Do they listen to the radio or television? What time of day and which programmes do they listen to? Which, if any, books, newspapers or magazines do they read? Do people put up pictures or calendars in their homes? What traditional media such as songs or drama do they enjoy? Which places do they pass that might be good places to put up posters?

Fig. 3.4 Questions to ask about your audience for planning communication

opinion leaders in your health education. Depending on the community, trust and *source-credibility* may come from:

- a person's natural position in the family community, e.g. village chief or elder;
- through their personal qualities or actions, e.g. a health worker who always comes out to help people even at night;
- qualifications and training;
- the extent to which the source shares characteristics such as age, culture, education, experiences with the receiver.

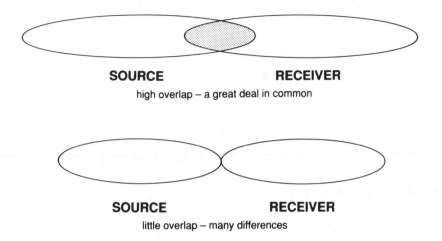

SOURCE   **RECEIVER**

high overlap – a great deal in common

SOURCE   **RECEIVER**

little overlap – many differences

Fig. 3.5   Source and receiver in communication

In which of the cases in Figure 3.5 do you think that communication will be more effective? A person from a similar background to the community is more likely to share the same language, ideas and motivations and thus be a more effective communicator. One of the main reasons for communication failure is when the source comes from a different background from the receiver and uses inappropriate message content and appeals.

This principle – that people who share similar backgrounds communicate better with each other – has important implications for health education. It explains why health workers who are strangers to the local community are not always effective in their health education work. Because of this, many health education programmes recruit field agents and volunteers from the community they are serving in.

Even if the field workers do not come from the local community, it is still possible to help them become closer to the community. The word *empathy* is used to describe the process by which a person learns to understand how others feel and think. Empathy is essential to becoming a good communicator. An important part of communication skill training is helping people to develop empathy with their communities. The best way to develop empathy is role-play which is described in Chapter 4. In role-play, you can try out situations and learn what it feels like to be a member of the community such as a mother having to find time to prepare oral rehydration therapy or to overcome opposition from the grandmother.

The communication message

The message consists of what is actually communicated including the actual appeals, words, pictures and sounds that you use to get the ideas across.

The nature of the advice given

A message will only be effective if the advice presented is relevant, appropriate, acceptable and put across in an understandable way. In deciding what advice to give, you will need to apply both an understanding of health and disease as well as the various influences on behaviour described in the previous chapter.

51

Fig. 3.6 Characteristics of good advice

The type of appeal

The appeal is the way we organise the content of the message to persuade or convince people. There is a tendency for many health education communications to use logical arguments that rely heavily on medical details. However, as shown here, many other approaches are possible.

Types of appeals in health communications

fear – a message may try to frighten people into action by emphasizing the serious outcome from not taking action. Symbols such as dying persons, coffins, grave stones, skulls may be used.

humour – the message is conveyed in a funny way such as a cartoon.

logical/factual appeal – emphasis in the message on conveying the need for action by giving facts, figures and information, e.g. on the causes of disease.

emotional appeal – attempts to convince people by arousing emotions, images and feelings rather than giving facts and figures, e.g. showing smiling babies, wealthy families with latrines, etc., associating the action with sex.

one-sided message – only presents the advantages of taking action and does not mention any possible disadvantages.

two-sided message – presents both the benefits and disadvantages ('pros and cons') of taking action.

positive appeals – communications that ask people to do something, e.g. breastfeed your child, build a latrine.

negative appeals – communications that ask people NOT to do something – i.e. do not bottle-feed your child, do not defaecate in the bush.

Not everyone responds in the same way to a message. What might persuade you might be quite different from what might persuade another person. For example what kinds of appeals do you think might convince each of the following: persons with little schooling; persons of a high educational level; children; and health workers?

Fear-appeal. Evidence suggests that mild fear can arouse interest, create concern and lead to change. However, too much fear can lead to people denying and

Fig. 3.7 Examples of appeals

rejecting the message. For example, health education on smoking in Britain used fear approaches of showing diseased lungs and descriptions of the harmful effects of smoking. This had little effect on smokers who built up a barrier of beliefs to deny the message and justify their smoking. Education on AIDS in many countries has involved fear-appeals including symbols of death such as skulls. With some people this has resulted in laughter and failure to take seriously the risk of AIDS; with others this approach has led to panic responses, stress and anxiety.

However, the use of fear is not simply one of whether it will persuade people to act. It involves ethical issues as well. Fear might be aroused but a person may not be able to take action to change – this can lead to considerable stress and anxiety. Many health educators feel that it is wrong to try to frighten people into action – unless there is clear evidence that benefits in health would result and that the means (i.e. enabling factors) are readily available to perform the action.

Humour. Humour is a very good way of attracting interest and attention. It can also serve a useful role to lighten the tension when dealing with serious subjects. Enjoyment and entertainment can result in highly-effective remembering and learning. However, humour does not always lead to changes in beliefs and attitudes. Humour is also very subjective – what one person finds funny another person may not.

Logical/factual compared with emotional appeals. A repeated observation from health education programmes throughout the world is that information on its own is usually not enough to change beliefs, attitudes and behaviour. Logical/factual arguments discussing disease patterns, parasite cycles and epidemiology will only carry weight with persons of a high educational level. Persons with less education will often be more convinced by simple emotional appeals from people they trust and stressing locally-held values such as motherhood, prestige, strength, etc.

Despite this, many health educators still feel that it is important to present some factual information because it allows people to make informed decisions. But it is important to be realistic about the limitations of just relying on facts to persuade people.

One-sided compared with two-sided messages. Presenting only one side of an argument may be effective if your audience will not be exposed to different views. However, if they are likely to hear opposing information, it can create suspicion that you are hiding something and not being honest. If there are some drawbacks to taking your advice – such as side-effects from a drug – it is better to be honest and admit them rather than let people find them out for themselves and then blame you for concealing them. Many health educators would also say that their main emphasis is not just to make people change behaviour but to help communities develop decision-making and problem-solving skills. Giving different points of view and helping them to distinguish the best actions to take is an important part of this process.

When you are face-to-face with individuals or groups it is easy to present both sides and make sure that the audience understands the issues. This is much more difficult in mass media such as radio, television and newspapers where the audience may only grasp part of the message or selectively pick up the points that they agree with. If you present both sides on the mass media you must test these messages carefully to make sure that the audience is not confused by receiving different points of view.

Positive and negative appeals. Negative appeals use terms such as 'avoid' or 'don't' to discourage people from performing harmful behaviours, e.g. 'don't bottlefeed', 'do not defaecate in the bush'. Most health educators agree that it is better to be positive and promote a beneficial behaviour, e.g. 'breast feed your baby', 'use a latrine'.

Formats

In theory, a message could use any of the five senses: sight, hearing, touch, taste and smell. However, the senses we mainly use in health communications are hearing and vision.

A great deal of information can be conveyed through sounds. Words can either be in spoken or written form and as songs. In addition to words, much information is conveyed through *non-verbal communication*. This includes gestures, hand-movements, direction of looking, tone of voice and appearance. A more detailed discussion of the important role that non-verbal communication plays in face-to-face communication is provided in Chapter 5.

In a book, information is conveyed in both the pictures and the words. You can use more than one format at a time: for example a health worker talking to a person and showing a leaflet or flip-chart would involve formats for face-to-face and leaflets described in Table 3.2.

Actual content of message

This includes the actual words, pictures, sounds that make up the communication and convey the appeals. In a radio programme the content would be a mix of: the advice given, wording, tone of voice, music. A poster would contain the basic appeal, pictures, words, photographs, symbols and colours.

In visual communications we can carry out a 'visual analysis' and analyze the content of a visual communication and specify:

• what is actually said; which words are used;

Table 3.2 Formats used in different communication methods

Face-to-face	spoken words
	non-verbal communication
	visual – real objects and models
	pictures/written words (when a visual aid is used)
Mass media	
radio	spoken words, non-verbal communication
television	spoken words, visual format
	non-verbal communication, written words
leaflets, books, newspapers	written words, visual pictures

- the type of letters used; whether capital letters (UPPER CASE) or small letters (lower case), lettering style, e.g. ordinary or *italics*;
- size of the actual letters;
- colour and printing method;
- the pictures used (illustrations), whether photographs (with or without backgrounds), or drawings (detailed, simple line drawings, or stylized drawings/cartoons);
- the size and colour of the pictures.

How does the message content influence attention?

Decisions such as whether to listen to one radio programme or another are deliberate ones. But others take place without conscious thought such as whether we happen to notice one poster out of many when we are going down a street or choose a particular book on a shelf.

A good example of the brain's ability to select information is the 'cocktail party phenomenon'. In a crowded room you can concentrate on listening to the person you are talking with and filter out the noise of all the other persons. But your ears and brain are still receiving all the other noises and if someone mentions something significant such as your own name you will notice – pay attention to – it.

It has been suggested by the psychologist Broadbent that the human brain acts as a filter (Figure 3.8). The brain processes the information it receives from the senses and decides what it will ignore and what it will pay attention to and interpret.

Sense organs (eyes and ears)	Mental filter	Interpretation
All light and sound waves received by eyes and ears.	Subconscious process selecting what information should be paid attention to.	Brain interprets information which is received.

Fig. 3.8 Broadbent Filter Model of selective attention

Think about what communications have attracted your attention recently and see if you can draw any lessons. What characteristics would draw your attention to each of the following: a magazine on a magazine stall; a radio programme; a poster on a wall with other posters? The factors that make communications attract attention fall into two main groups: physical and motivational characteristics.

Physical characteristics that attract attention include:
- size, e.g. of the whole poster – we are more likely to notice a large poster or book than a small one; size of letters – large letters on a poster, title words;
- intensity – bold headings in a sentence, poster;
- high-pitched sounds, e.g. the cry of a baby, police sirens, loud noises;
- colour – primary colours such as reds, yellows, orange;
- pictures – photographs and drawings.

Motivational characteristics that attract attention include:
- novelty – unusual features, unfamiliar and surprising objects;
- interest – interests/felt needs of audience and perceived relevance to audience – people look at things they are interested in and want to know something about;
- deeper motivations – appeals to motivations and drives of audience, e.g. sex;
- entertainment and humour.

The design of a poster, including colour, size, lettering and use of pictures can increase its likelihood of gaining attention and being noticed. Communications which attract attention are also those which deal with subjects that the target group *want* to know something about, i.e. which fit in with their felt needs and interests. Another way of attracting attention is by including something unusual in the communication that arouses interest. You can include unusual objects in exhibitions, incorporate drama in a public meeting, have an unusual picture on a poster, begin a radio programme with an attention-getting sound.

Many health communications have failed because they have been boring, dull and emphasize medical facts. You should remember that people like to be entertained – and that, just because you are interested in the subject, it does not mean that others will be. You should explore ways of making your educational work interesting and fun. For example, if you are making a radio programme, you can make it more interesting by using a variety of formats including music, drama, interviews, quizzes, etc. You can read more about entertainment and media in Chapters 7 and 8.

It is also important to hold attention in face-to-face communication and teaching sessions so your audience listen carefully. In the next chapter you will see how an important function of learning aids is to arouse the interest of a group.

Perception and understanding

Problems in understanding take place when the person receiving the message misinterprets the various words, pictures and non-verbal signals that make up the message. It is not difficult to understand how misunderstandings take place when the message is in an unfamiliar language. It is also obvious that the writing in a leaflet or poster will not be understood by a person who cannot read and write. However, even when persons speak the same language, there can be problems in communication – for example, if unfamiliar or technical words are used. It is also easy to come to the wrong conclusions about the meaning of looks, gestures and tones of voice that make up non-verbal communication.

Because of the need to communicate to illiterate persons, health educators often put emphasis on using pictures rather than words in posters and leaflets. It was thought that pictures are a universal language. However, pictures themselves contain a 'visual language' with special ways for showing distance, direction, motion and even emotions such as happiness, and strength.

A picture is drawn on a flat sheet of paper but the real world is solid. A picture can only show one part of an object whereas in the real world we can walk around an object to see many different views. Drawings usually simplify objects and have less detail. The real world is in colour whereas the high expense of colour printing means that pictures in books are often in black and white. People who have not had much experience of looking at pictures can easily misinterpret the message. *Visual literacy* is the term used for a person's familiarity with interpreting pictures.

Some of the well-known studies of visual literacy have been carried out in Kenya, Nepal, Lesotho, Zambia and Ghana. These have involved showing a range of pictures to samples of the community to find out which ones they could correctly identify. Some of the kinds of pictures that were not understood include: stylized diagrams, e.g. line drawings, 'stick men', silhouettes and use of shading to show light and shadows; biological diagrams such as life cycles, pictures of organs, anatomical drawings, parts of body; pictures showing emotions such as happiness, strength and sickness; pictures using artist's conventions for showing movement, relative size of objects, as well as relative distances (horizons, converging lines, etc.); symbols such as $+$, $-$, $\times$, %, $\vee$, $\rightarrow$; use of colours to show feelings, e.g. red for danger. Some examples of different pictures used in these studies are shown in Figure 3.9.

These visual literacy studies tell us a great deal about the psychological processes involved in perception. When people hear or see something they try to give it a meaning that 'makes sense' to them. Perception thus involves *guessing* at the meaning from the information available. If not enough information is available in a picture, the guess may be wrong and the picture may not be understood. In radio programmes there is often the background noise of other programmes

Fig. 3.9 Visual literacy styles

which can make it difficult to make out the words. A similar problem can be found in pictures when there is too much information, distracting background and unnecessary details.

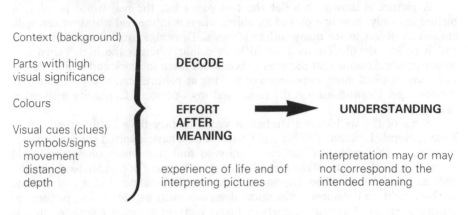

Fig. 3.10 The process of visual perception

Perception does not happen instantly but is a process over a short time period (see Figure 3.10). A person will take in the different information (or 'clues') and arrive at an interpretation. We can even measure this with machines that follow eye movements. A person will first look at the striking or unusual features which attract attention and then take in further details until the interpretation is reached. In trying to guess the meaning of a part of a picture, a person will take into account the background. If the picture is not immediately obvious, the person will choose an interpretation that fits with the details that caught his/her attention in the background.

Perception depends on a person's experience. You will find difficulty recognizing and giving a name to something that you have never seen before. For example, a study in Kenya found that a person seeing a picture of a cupboard who had never seen a real cupboard before was not able to identify it and instead identified it as something else.

Problems of misunderstanding can be particularly serious with mass media, with its lack of immediate feedback to check if correct understanding has taken place. Misunderstanding of communication is more likely to take place when the artist, radio producer or communication designer comes from a different background from that of the target audience. This is especially so when the audience is rural and of low educational status and the communication planners are urban, highly-educated and from different cultural backgrounds. The best way of overcoming this cultural distance between the communication planners and the community is to find ways of involving the community in the production of the materials. It is also important to pre-test the prototypes (first versions) carefully before they are broadcast or printed.

As education and access to printed materials increases, so also should people become more familiar with interpreting pictures. A recent study by UNICEF in Nepal, *Rethinking Visual Literacy*, showed that, with a small teaching input, it is not difficult to learn to understand pictures. I have summarized the findings of a number of studies on visual communication to produce the guidelines shown. Even with these guidelines it is essential to *pre-test* any communication that is used.

58

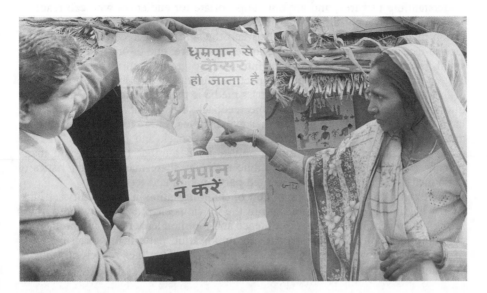

Fig. 3.11 Pre-testing of posters in India

Guidelines to using pictures

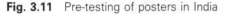

1. Make details accurate and of objects familiar to the target audience.
2. Avoid distracting details.
3. If you use colour make it accurate.
4. Distortions in size (e.g. enlargements) should be avoided.
5. Show complete objects – especially parts of the body.
6. Show objects from familiar angles (be careful of cross-sections and anatomical drawings).
7. Be careful when using perspective (showing relative distance).
8. Use signs and symbols that are understood by the target audience.
9. Be careful when using sequences of pictures as it can easily cause confusion.
10. Single communications should not contain more than one message.
11. Always pre-test with samples of your intended audience.

Channel

This is also sometimes referred to as the *communication method*. There are two main groups of methods: face-to-face ('interpersonal') and mass media. Each channel provides opportunities to use a different combination of *formats* (see Table 3.2).

Mass media include broadcast media (radio and television) as well as print media (newspapers, books, leaflets and wall posters) and are described in more detail in Chapter 8. Television involves both a sound and a visual dimension. Radio involves sound only. Radio-ownership is high in many countries which makes it a particularly valuable medium where literacy is low. Print media such as newspapers, books and leaflets, which use the written word, also require familiarity in understanding pictures, and are only appropriate for audiences who can read.

Face-to-face or interpersonal methods include all those forms of communication involving direct interaction between the source and receiver. Examples of face-to-face methods with increasing audience size are: one-to-one and counselling; small group (less than 12 persons); intermediate group/lecture (between 12 and 30); and large group lecture /public meeting (more than 30). The main advantage of face-to-face communication over mass media is that it creates opportunities for questions, discussion, participation and feedback. It is possible to check that you have been understood and give further explanations. However, as the size of the group increases, it is more difficult to have feedback and discussion. In large groups and public meetings usually only a small number take part and many persons feel shy speaking out. So public meetings share many characteristics of mass media in that they involve limited participation and feedback.

We can look at the direction of flow of communication in community settings. At the beginning of this chapter and in the previous chapter you saw how it was important to consider sources of influence and 'opinion leadership' in families and communities. You can represent the communication pattern or 'social network' in a community by a diagram such as Figure 3.12. The lines represent a line of communication between two people.

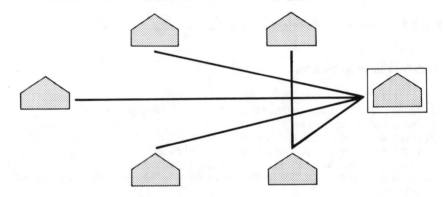

Fig. 3.12 Communication networks in communities

Analyzing the flow of communication in a community ('sociometric' analysis) will show if there are 'opinion leaders'. They may be elders, shopkeepers or just people who have acquired some influence or importance. They form the *internal communication system* within a community that you need to understand before planning any health education activities. If you can obtain the full support of the opinion leaders then it should be easy to convince a community to take up health-promoting innovations. If the opinion leaders are against you it will be extremely difficult to work in a community.

The expansion of printed media, radio and television that is taking place makes it easy to forget that most traditional forms of communication involve face-to-face or *oral communication*. Traditional or 'popular' media such as drama, singing, dancing, storytelling and proverb-telling may exist in your community. Community gatherings, religious meetings and ceremonies can provide opportunities for health education. This provides an example of the approach of 'starting where people are at' rather than imposing forms of communication that are unfamiliar to the community. Chapter 7 describes how you can mobilize popular media for health education and health promotion.

Comparison of mass media and face-to-face communication methods

Mass media are the best methods for rapid spread of simple information and facts to a large population at low cost. If the advice is realistic (see Figure 3.6) and the message pre-tested, the message can be accurately transmitted without the distortions that can sometimes take place when we rely on word-of-mouth.

However, as mass media are broadcast to the whole population, they are not a good method for selectively reaching specific groups, e.g. grandmothers or teenagers. It is difficult to make the message appropriate to the special situation of local communities, whose problems and needs may be different from the rest of the country. Even if a person hears something on the radio and wishes to change, he or she may be pressurized against change by those around them. Furthermore, health education often involves influencing beliefs and attitudes and developing problem-solving skills. For these more difficult objectives, participatory learning methods involving group discussion, sharing of experience and problem-solving exercises will be more effective.

Table 3.3 Main characteristics of mass media and face-to-face channels

Characteristics	Mass media	Face-to-face
speed to cover large population	rapid	slow
accuracy and lack of distortion	high accuracy	easily distorted
ability to select particular audience	difficult to select audience	can be highly selective
direction	one-way	two-way
ability to respond to local needs of specific communities	only provides non-specific information	can fit to local need
feed-back	only indirect feedback from surveys	direct feedback possible
main effect	increased/knowledge awareness	changes in attitudes and behaviour; problem-solving skills

Face-to-face methods are slower for spreading information in a population because of the need to mobilize fieldworkers and travel to the different communities to hold meetings. However, the opportunity to ask the audience questions and obtain feedback gives face-to-face methods a powerful advantage. It is possible to contact specific groups, make the advice relevant to their special needs and develop problem-solving skills and community participation. Feedback makes it possible to check for misunderstandings and give clarification and explain particular points.

The communications researcher Everett Rogers has reviewed many studies of how new practices or 'innovations' spread or 'diffuse' within communities. He suggests that adoption of new practices such as using latrines or oral rehydration therapy takes place through stages: initially a person becomes aware of the existence of the new practice; he/she may become interested, then decide to try it out and, if satisfied, adopt it. Rogers' *Communication of Innovations Theory* suggests that mass media can provide the necessary background information for change but are usually insufficient on their own to change behaviour – especially if you are trying to change long-established customs. Most health behaviour-changes will require face-to-face communication using community-based approaches, home-visiting, involvement of opinion leaders and community participation.

Fig. 3.13   Influence of communication methods on adoption of innovations

Mostly, it is not simply a case of either mass media or interpersonal methods. A well-planned programme will involve a carefully chosen *mix* of both approaches which exploits their different advantages. Figure 3.15 shows a communication strategy for an oral rehydration programme in Honduras. This combined different approaches with activities timed to coincide with the seasonal peaks in diarrhoea. Radio reinforces the face-to-face communication by field workers and printed materials have been produced to support the programme.

Fig. 3.14   Choice of methods

Fig. 3.15 Communication strategy for promotion of oral rehydration in Honduras

Deciding what communication method to use

Choice of communication method and supporting learning aids will depend on what you are trying to achieve, the nature of your audience and what resources are at your disposal. Some of the questions you will need to ask to make this decision are listed below. The starting point for selection of media should be your analysis of what you are trying to convey. Are you going to try to change a belief – and is it a weakly-held one or a strongly-held one rooted in culture or experience, as described in the previous chapter? What type of learning will you be trying to promote? You should read the section on learning in the next chapter that will show how you can separate-out the learning involved into simple and complex facts, skills and attitudes.

Each method provides different opportunities for formats including visual, sounds, verbal and non-verbal communication (see Table 3.2). If you want to help a person to recognize a child's fast breathing at the onset of a severe respiratory infection you will need a medium with the dimension of sound. If you want to show someone what a condom or an improved latrine *looks* like you will need a method which has a visual dimension.

In addition, you will also have to consider practical considerations of cost, complexity and feasibility of use. If you are working in a local community you are unlikely to have access to mass media such as radio or newspapers. You may not have any fieldworkers at your disposal so have no choice but to concentrate on methods that do not require staffing.

A useful guide to planning your health education is to start with simpler methods such as mass media such as radio, leaflets and posters and see if they are effective. Only if the simple methods do not work should you move on to more expensive methods involving extensive use of fieldworkers and other interpersonal methods. Short-term approaches can be accompanied by longer-term strategies such as working through schools and the workplace.

Criteria for selecting methods

Your 'learning' objectives
Do you need to convey simple facts, complex information, problem-solving skills, practical manual ('psycho-motor') skills, attitudes and behaviour change? (See Chapter 4 for further discussion of learning.)

Other programme considerations
Will you need a visual dimension, e.g. a picture, to explain your point? Is sound necessary?
How accepting is the community of new ideas? Will they be resistant to your advice?
How urgent is your time scale? Is it a short- or long-term priority?
Do you want to develop community participation?

Characteristics of the audience
What are the characteristics of the audience that will affect choice of methods? e.g. age, experience of life, education and literacy level, previous exposure to pictures; ownership of radio/TVs, listening, watching and reading habits; familiarity with different media, traditional communication methods already in use? (See also audience characteristics on page 52.)

Characteristics of different methods
How much will the different methods cost, including initial costs and operating and maintenance?
How many staff and what level of skill are involved in using the method? What field

requirements will affect the use of the equipment, e.g. for electricity, blackout, storage and transport?

Costs

availability of funds for initial purchase, spare parts and maintenance

need for electricity, black-out

need for/availability of trained staff for media production, maintenance and implementation

the need for trained fieldworkers in the community to implement the method

---

Summary of the communication planning process

Communication planning involves two main groups of decisions: what are the aims of the communication and who should be the target group? Making these decisions involves the application of ideas introduced in the first two chapters of this book.

The second set of decisions has been the subject of this chapter – the choice of source, messages and channels required to promote the desired changes.

1. A communication can go through a series of stages before it can have an impact on improvement of health. These stages are: reaching the senses; gaining attention; understanding; acceptance of the message; and change in behaviour. A detailed understanding of the characteristics of the community is needed to make decisions about the best source, message and channel.
2. Messages should be pre-tested to make sure that they will attract attention, be correctly understood, acceptable and relevant to the problem. This is especially important with mass media when the message has to stand on its own and there is no opportunity to check for misunderstanding.
3. Communication should be evaluated to find out if it has achieved each of the six stages from reaching the senses to improvement of health. Lessons learnt from evaluation should be used to design better programmes.
4. Conclusions from Chapter 3 can be combined with the basic principles of communication theory introduced in this chapter to produce the guidelines for effective health communications listed here.

Characteristics of effective health communication

Promotes actions that are realistic and feasible within the constraints faced by the community.

Builds on ideas, concepts and practices that people already have.

Repeated and reinforced over time using different methods.

Adaptable, and uses existing channels of communication – for example, songs, drama and storytelling.

Entertaining and attracts community's attention.

Uses clear simple language with local expressions and emphasizes short-term benefits of action.

Provides opportunities for dialogue and discussion to allow learner-participation and feedback on understanding and implementation.

Uses demonstrations to show the benefits of adopting practices.

---

4. The effective teacher

If I only hear it, I forget it.
When people just sit and listen to someone else talk, they will not learn very much.
If I hear and see it, I remember it.
When people see for themselves what things look like and how they work, they will learn more than if they just listened to someone else talk about it.
If I hear, see and do it, I know it.
When people not only hear and see, but actually do, make and discover things for themselves, they will learn the most.

Teaching and learning are essential to most health education and health promotion activities. Training is really another word for teaching. It is often applied to the process of introducing the community or other fieldworkers to new ideas, information and skills – either in their initial training or later as part of their *continuing* education.

People can learn in many different ways. This chapter will deal with learning that takes place through organized face-to-face situations in groups – either small or large. It will build on concepts of communication introduced in the previous chapter as well as set the scene for the discussion of face-to-face communication in the next chapter. It will help you to:

1. Decide what to include in your teaching – i.e. set the objectives.
2. Choose teaching methods and learning aids.
3. Plan training courses.

Deciding what to include in your teaching

You may only have a few hours available with a particular group, or as much as a month. In either case you will have to decide what are the most important topics to cover and set priority objectives for your teaching. Objectives are precise statements of what you intend to achieve through your planned learning activities. Setting objectives will help you to decide: what to include in the learning activities; what learning methods to use, and how to assess the effectiveness of your teaching activities. A *curriculum* is a set of objectives with details of the learning methods by which you will reach those objectives.

The initial reason for planning some teaching is usually a need that has arisen in your work. For example, you may have to update fieldworkers on a new disease such as AIDS, introduce new skills such as preparation of oral rehydration solution or preparation and use of a learning aid such as flip-charts.

In planning training we begin by specifying the behaviours – sometimes called 'competences' – that the fieldworkers must be able to perform in order to contribute to the health education programme. This list of desired actions is often called a *job description* or *job specification* and forms the basis of identifying training needs, e.g. Figure 4.1. Preparing a job description and resulting curriculum involves asking the questions in Figure 4.2.

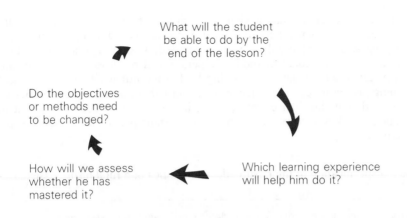

What will the student
be able to do by the
end of the lesson?

Do the objectives
or methods need
to be changed?

How will we assess
whether he has
mastered it?

Which learning experience
will help him do it?

Fig. 4.1 Curriculum design and objective setting for training programmes

- What do you require the community or fieldworker to *do* to implement the programme you have planned? These actions should be written out as a detailed job specification.
- What activities in the job specification is the person already able to undertake?
- What activities in the job specification will the person require training to be able to undertake?
- What does the person require to successfully carry out those activities?

Fig. 4.2 Questions to ask in preparing a job specification

You can prepare a job description by: studying the problem and possible solutions; observing successful fieldworkers and the methods they have used; consulting other persons with relevant experience. Your proposed job description should be realistic and feasible.

Many fieldworkers already have job descriptions that form the basis for their conditions of employment. The job specification that you develop for planning a training programme will usually be more detailed. It should describe the kinds of decisions and educational methods the person will be expected to use in their work. You can then evaluate the training by finding out whether, at the end of the teaching programme, the participants can actually undertake the activities you have specified. (In the final chapter, you will also see that decisions about job specifications for key fieldworkers form an important part of the process of programme planning.)

Sample job specification of the health education duties of a rural health assistant

---

1. Carry out a community diagnosis to determine: health education needs; influences on behaviour; opinion leaders and social networks.
2. Carry out one-to-one health education with a range of persons on topics such as water supply, sanitation, food hygiene and nutrition.
3. Carry out group health education with community groups.
4. Give health education talks at public meetings.
5. Advise teachers on school health education and give talks to pupils in classes.
6. Advise families on setting up of kitchen gardens for promotion of nutrition.
7. Supervise health education activities of community health workers.
8. Prepare health education demonstration programmes on water supply and sanitation.
9. Work as a part of a team with other personnel in the promotion of primary health care and integrated rural development.
10. Collect local data for planning and evaluating health education programmes.

Task analysis and specifying the kinds of learning

The kinds of learning involving intellectual or thinking tasks are called 'cognitive' learning. These are distinguished from 'affective' learning which covers emotions, feelings, attitudes and values. The different kinds of learning include:

- *knowledge*   facts, specific information;
- *skills*   'thinking' decision-making and problem-solving skills; communication skills, e.g. one-to-one and group; psychomotor skills, e.g. handling, mixing;
- *attitudes*   feelings, emotions, values.

The word 'know' is used in a vague way in everyday speech. Consider the following: knowing the life-cycle of hookworm, knowing how to design a sanitation programme, knowing how to build a latrine and knowing how to talk to a community meeting. These are each quite different kinds of learning and are respectively: factual knowledge, decision-making skills, psychomotor skills and communication skills.

Each activity in a job description will require a different combination of knowledge, skills and attitudes. The term *task analysis* is used for the process of analysing the actions in a job description to determine the kinds of learning involved.

68

Knowledge and decision-making skills

A useful way of separating types of cognitive learning was suggested by the educationist Bloom. He suggests that there are different levels of cognitive learning. These range from simpler *'lower-order'* cognitive skills such as factual knowledge and comprehension to more complex 'higher-order' skills such as application, analysis, synthesis and evaluation which can be called problem-solving skills.

Knowledge is the simplest level and includes knowledge of terms, facts and principles. Examples are:

> Listing the causes of diarrhoea.
> Describing the ways in which diarrhoea can be prevented.
> Describing how bacteria can cause infection.

Some facts can be simple to learn. Others, such as the life-cycle of a parasite are more difficult, especially if it is an unfamiliar subject. Teaching facts involves the following steps: relating the information to previous knowledge; presenting the information logically in a step-by-step fashion; using visual aids to explain relationships and avoiding presenting too much information in one session and causing overload. Face-to-face contact is helpful for explaining more complicated facts as it is possible to ask questions to check understanding. If the facts are simple and the educational level of your audience is sufficiently high, you can use distance-learning methods such as a newsletter or books.

More complex *'higher-order'* thinking skills involve application of knowledge, interpretation of facts, theories, problem-solving and decision-making; these usually require some knowledge first. Some examples are given below of thinking skills with more difficult higher-order ones given at the end of the list.

> Interpretation of facts, relationships or theories.
> Separating preventive behaviours into primary, secondary and tertiary.
> Interpretation of existing data, such as determining the health problems of communities from clinic data.
> Choosing a balanced diet from the foods provided.
> Using a growth chart to assess whether an infant is at risk of developing malnutrition.
> Analyzing the influences on a person's health behaviour.
> Writing a radio script to encourage mothers to breastfeed.
> Designing an educational programme for the prevention of diarrhoea.
> Deriving a theory to explain relationships, e.g. construction of a model to explain why people do not use health services.
> Evaluation of a health education plan for the promotion of breastfeeding.

Decision-making skills are taught by: first providing the necessary basic information; then demonstrating the skills with worked-out examples; and following this by allowing the students to practise making the decisions in realistic situations such as case studies, role-plays and field exercises. More time and effort are required to learn those complex skills at the end of the above list than the simpler ones given earlier. For example: knowledge about vitamins and food tables is required in order to practise the more advanced skill of calculating the vitamin content of a meal; knowledge about the advantages and disadvantages of different sources of water is required to practise the more complex skill of choosing an appropriate water source for a community.

Communication skills

Communication involves a combination of *decision-making skills* and *communication skills* including:

Choosing objectives.
Deciding actual content of advice, i.e. what to say.
Deciding which learning aids to use.
Ability to speak clearly and sufficiently loud to be heard.
Ability to listen, ask questions, promote discussion.
Use of non-verbal communication including gestures, eye contact, tone of voice and posture to establish rapport, show concern and encourage responses.

The best way of teaching communication skills is: first, to demonstrate good communication to the learners; and then let everyone in the training group practise the skills with each other in role-plays. For example, you can ask someone to give a talk to the others who act as villagers and respond. Afterwards, everyone can discuss how well the talk was done. You can give the audience a checklist like the one below to judge how well the communication was carried out.

Was it interesting?
Was it clear?
Were the visual aids used well?
Was there good use of questions?
Was everyone encouraged to participate in discussion?

After everyone has had a chance to practise the communication skill, you can have a general discussion to bring out main points. You should encourage a friendly atmosphere of helpful criticism and explain that we can only learn by making mistakes and learning from them. However, if you feel that your students may be sensitive to criticism, you can give individual feedback afterwards. If a video camera is available, it is a good idea to record the communication exercise so that they can see themselves afterwards. We all have mannerisms such as moving about, jangling keys, scratching noses, using favourite phrases and we often only realise it when we actually see ourselves! Once everyone has had a chance to try out the communication in a safe and friendly environment, you can let them try it out in a real situation with the community. This could involve asking them to teach a class with you observing and giving some feedback afterwards on how it went.

Psycho-motor skills

Psycho-motor skills involve learning how to perform manual operations such as threading film projectors, using drawing instruments, putting on a condom and giving injections. Often they are accompanied by decisions. For example, in addition to the skill of mixing oral rehydration solution, a mother would need to be able to decide how much and when to give the solution to her child. The decision-making and psycho-motor skills can be taught separately.

Demonstration and providing opportunities to practise in pretended and real-life situations are the best ways of teaching psycho-motor skills. For example, you could ask students to: put a condom onto a model of a penis; mix up oral rehydration solution and give it to a baby; add some oil to a weaning food and mix to the right consistency; build a latrine.

Attitudes

Attitudes involve a person's feelings towards something or someone. Attitudes are difficult to define and, because of this, are often left out of training programmes. However, it's not enough teaching someone facts and skills. Whether the training is taken seriously and put into practice will usually depend on his or her attitudes. Some examples of important attitudes are:

Feeling that the topic of the training is important and should be put into practice.
Realising the importance of making follow-up visits.
Taking care and being accurate when measuring the weight of a child.
Being prepared to work among disadvantaged and poor people.
Being patient and prepared to listen to and respect the community.
Taking care to properly prepare one's health education.

Many people question whether it is actually possible to 'teach' attitudes such as commitment to working among poor people. They point to the importance of selection of people who already are motivated and show the necessary attitudes. However, there are several ways in which you can influence attitudes. One way is to provide opportunities for participants in your training programmes to discuss the importance of the attitudes involved.

Another way of developing attitudes is by personal example. Students often see their teachers as 'role models'. If you are trying to develop attitudes of sensitivity, commitment to work, thoroughness, accuracy, attention to detail, planning of work, one of the best ways is to set an example by your own personal behaviour. People will also be more likely to develop attitudes if they see that those attitudes are recognized and encouraged by their supervisors and employers.

In health education training we are often trying to develop respect and understanding of other people's point of view – empathy. A powerful method for developing empathy is to ask people to act out a situation in the community in a role-play, e.g. a woman receiving inappropriate health education on child-feeding. Through role-play, the person can experience what it is like to be another person. Role-play is discussed in more detail later in this chapter.

Identifying types of learning

Now that the different kinds of learning have been described, you can practise with the example below. Look at the different activities in the list and identify types of learning, separating them into simple knowledge, skills (thinking, communication and psycho-motor) and attitudes. Check your answers against the correct ones. Once you are confident that you can distinguish different kinds of learning you can apply the checklist provided, to help you plan your teaching.

Exercise on recognizing different kinds of learning

---

1. Nurse knowing how to make a flipchart.
2. Village health worker being able to list the advantages of breastfeeding.
3. The ability to demonstrate to mothers how to give oral rehydration therapy solution.
4. Clinic nurses wanting to spend time promoting latrines.

5. Nurses taking blood pressure.
6. Village health worker being able to list the sources of vitamin A.
7. Nurse choosing a balanced diet from available foods.
8. Nurses knowing the procedures for referral of TB patients.
9. Nurse deciding when to refer a patient to hospital.
10. Nurse being able to write down the different stages of the life cycle of the malaria parasite.
11. Nurse being able to plan how to prevent malaria in her community.
12. Nurse wanting to spend time in the community promoting malaria spraying.
13. Health assistant being aware of the services provided by the health education department.
14. Health assistant being aware of the importance of doing health education.

Answers (1) decision-making (content of flipchart) as well as psycho-motor (how to draw, bind pages); (2) factual knowledge; (3) factual knowledge about ORT, psycho-motor skills in preparation of ORT, communication skills; (4) attitude; (5) psycho-motor skills and well as decision-making; (6) factual knowledge; (7) factual knowledge of nutrients and sources of foods, decision-making as to choosing combinations; (8) factual knowledge of procedures; (9) knowledge of procedures as well as decision-making skill of deciding in a given case whether to refer); (10) factual learning; (11) decision-making skill; (12) attitude; (13) factual knowledge; (14) attitude.

A checklist for analyzing the learning components of your programme

What information should the audience know by the end of the session?
Either: simple facts *or* more complicated facts?
What problem-solving or decision-making skills will they need to acquire?
What communication skills do they need to acquire?
What manual (psycho-motor) skills should they have by the end of the session?
What attitudes should they have by the end of the session?

Setting objectives

Learning objectives are statements of the learning to be achieved by the end of the teaching session. They form the basis for planning the content of the learning activities and for evaluation of the outcome. Learning objectives should specify:

- The exact learning required; WHAT is to change and by HOW MUCH.
- How the change will be measured, i.e. test conditions.
- The time over which the learning should take place.

The activities in a job description can form the overall objectives for a training programme. However, it is also helpful to set objectives for each type of learning needed to perform an activity.

An objective should be measurable. Psycho-motor skills such as handling objects or communication skills (see below) are not difficult to measure, as they can be directly observed. However changes in knowledge, thinking and attitudes are more difficult because they take place within a person's mind and are not directly observable. We can only measure them by expressing them as actions – or *behavioural objectives*. This involves asking people to carry out actions such as to give opinions, describe situations, answer questions and undertake tests. Some examples of behavioural objectives are given here.

Examples of behavioural objectives

By the end of the session the participants:
on being asked, will be able to list correctly the different stages of the life-cycle of malaria (*knowledge*);
on being taken to a house, will be able to choose the best location for a latrine (*decision-making*);
in a test situation, will be able to use a flannelgraph to encourage learner participation in a small-group teaching session (*communication skill*);
on being given a pencil, ruler and paper will be able to enlarge a picture using the 'squaring up' method (*psycho-motor*); and
on being given data and a growth chart, will take care to enter data correctly on to a growth chart and recognise what follow-up advice is needed for the mother (*attitude/decision-making*).

Some people are critical of using measurable objectives to plan and evaluate training activities. They feel that it can leave out changes in participants that are important but difficult to measure such as development of confidence, self-reliance and thinking skills – these are sometimes called personal growth. It also reinforces a 'top-down' approach which ignores the importance of the individual in deciding his or her own learning needs and outcomes. The critics of behavioural objectives would argue that the actual *process* of learning is as important as achieving particular outcomes.

Fig. 4.3 We need to promote effective teaching and learning

73

However, a reply to this criticism is that if we cannot measure the purpose of the learning, it's because we don't really know what we are trying to do! It would then be impossible to plan the programme or find out afterwards if we have been successful. In the past, training programmes have over-emphasized learning facts and we need to pay more attention to attitudes as well as higher-order cognitive learning processes such as decision-making and problem-solving. Also, we must recognize that training activities should not only concentrate on acquiring specific skills, but also include broader outcomes such as personal growth and the development of self-reliance. Chapter 6 will take up this discussion further when it considers the problem of setting objectives for community partici-pation programmes and Chapter 11 will also look at objectives for programme planning and evaluation.

Some guidelines for promotion of learning

Once you have undertaken the task analysis and identified the different kinds of learning you wish to promote, you can begin to choose your teaching strategies. Much attention has been paid by educational psychologists to examining ways in which people learn and a summary of some of the lessons learned is given here.

Guidelines for effective teaching and learning

- People learn better if the information you present is linked to their experiences and builds on what they already know. Always ask questions at the beginning to find out what people know, think and feel about the topic.
- Your audience will only pay attention to you if the content of your teaching is relevant to what they want to know about, is put across in an interesting way and uses a variety of teaching styles.
- Complicated information should be introduced step-by-step in a logical, organized way. Learning can be helped by well-chosen visual aids. Essential information can be on a handout and the time saved used for discussion.
- Take care not to overload your students with too many new ideas in one session as there is a limit to the amount of information that can be absorbed at one sitting. Try to use a range of teaching approaches such as talks, discussion, exercises and active learning methods. Build in frequent breaks between sessions where people can relax and stretch their legs. Twenty minutes at a time is probably the most people can concentrate.
- Information presented in a teaching session is quickly forgotten. Some further input, either by the student's own reading or reminders by the teacher, is needed for the information to be retained in long-term memory.
- Your audience may have enjoyed themselves and express appreciation but may not have learnt anything! The only way in which you can find out whether learning has taken place is by obtaining some feedback – either asking questions or observing their performance to see if they have improved.
- You should provide opportunities for your students to practise their newly-acquired skills in a safe, friendly and tolerant environment where they can make mistakes and receive helpful criticism without feeling threatened.
- People learn better if they are allowed to discover principles for themselves and activities are built into the learning process. Use active methods as follows:
  more active methods include: practice in real situations with supervision, practice in class situation, e.g. role-play; and discussion.
  less active methods: observing a drama or demonstration, looking at pictures; written examples, paper-and-pencil exercises; individual reading.

SUMMARY
Active learning: make students think and apply the knowledge through a task
Be clear: use visual aids, speak clearly, use simple language
Make it meaningful: explain in advance what you are going to teach; explain all new
   words and ideas; relate what you teach to student's lives and work; give
   examples; summarize main points at end.
Encourage participation: stimulate discussion and involve the group in the learning.
Ensure mastery: check understanding and competence reached.
Give feedback: tell the learners what their progress is.

Participatory learning

A serious criticism of many health education programmes is that they rely too
much on traditional formal teaching methods where the audience is passive and
simply listens. More emphasis is now placed on *participatory learning methods* and
dialogue such as small-group teaching, simulations, case studies, group exercises
and role-play. Participatory learning methods have many advantages. The participants are active and not passive so they are more likely to remember what was
introduced during the session. They draw from their own experience. They are
allowed to discover principles for themselves and can develop problem-solving
skills. Participatory learning methods are especially relevant for those who did
not do well at school. Other advantages of this approach are:

- it makes people think for themselves and be less dependent on you;
- it gives people greater pride in what they can do for themselves;
- you can discover the beliefs and practices of people in the community;
- it creates a close feeling between you and your group;
- it shows your interest and respect for the opinions of the community;
- it also makes health education more fun!

Fig. 4.4 Leading a discussion

One reason some people don't use participatory learning methods is shortage of time. A useful tip is to provide as much information as possible as handouts or a handbook. You can use the time saved for explaining difficult points, discussing important issues and introducing participatory learning methods.

Many people prefer giving a lecture and feel uncomfortable with the freer approach involved in a participatory learning situation. Sometimes they are worried that they will be asked questions that they can't answer. They can have problems getting a discussion going or dealing with individuals who dominate the class. If your audience is used to formal talks, they may feel shy about offering opinions and resistant to participatory methods. They may complain that you are not providing enough facts. Guidelines on leading a discussion are given below and more hints on working with groups are given in the next chapter.

---

1. Seating people in a circle around you is best for discussions. In a circle, there is no 'head' and so there is no 'tail' and everyone is equal. Sitting in a 'U' shape is the next best.
2. Tell your audience at the start that they will all be taking part in a health talk. Emphasize that you will NOT be doing all the talking.
3. Begin with easy questions. If you will be discussing more than one subject, begin with what you think people will be more free to talk about. This builds up people's confidence.
4. If you ask a question and no one answers, ask it again, using slightly different words.
5. Don't give up if answers are slow in coming. It will take people time to 'warm up' to this new way of learning.
6. Always respond with enthusiasm to any answer. Praise the people who answer, even if the answer is wrong: 'Thank you for your thoughts', 'That's interesting'; and 'Good for you for speaking up'.
7. Be sure to look around at everyone in the group. It is easy to look at only the one or two people who are answering all the questions and this discourages the others.
8. If someone asks you a question, a good way of keeping the discussion going is to direct the question back to the group: 'That's a very good question, Mrs Sharma. What do you think, Mrs Mthembu?'
9. The best discussions are short and leave people wishing for more. After an hour or so our minds begin to wander and not much learning can take place.
10. Practice makes perfect! Before you lead the real discussion, it is very helpful to practise. Ask some of your family and friends to sit around and pretend that they are the people you will be speaking to. Ask them the same questions you will be asking your 'real audience', to find out what their response is.

Role-play

Role-play is the use of drama in which people act out situations for themselves in order to acquire communication and problem-solving skills and understand situations. Role-plays can vary in length between an extended session lasting a whole day to a ten-minute activity within a training class.

Role-play can help us learn more about ourselves and why we behave as we do. Role-play can also help us to learn more about other people and their motivations. We can explore events from different points of view and develop empathy for communities. For example, men can act out the role of women and thus gain an understanding of the difficulties that they face in putting into practice health education messages.

Role-play is a very direct way of learning; you are given a role and have to think and speak immediately without detailed planning. Learning takes place through active experience; it is not passive. Role-play can be used to explore events that have already happened or which might happen. It uses situations that the members of the group are likely to find themselves in during their lives. It gives group members the chance to consider different ways of responding within those situations. Some people find it easier to explain an experience through acting it out rather than reporting it or writing it down. Some examples of role-play activities are given here.

Examples of role-play activities used in training

Ask a person to get into a wheelchair and move around a building to develop an understanding of what it feels like to be disabled.

Assign one person the role of a fieldworker and let the rest take on the roles of different members of a community. Have the fieldworker try to persuade the community to adopt a health practice, e.g. building latrines. After ten to fifteen minutes, stop the role-play and have a discussion about how successful (or unsuccessful!) the fieldworker was and how the approach could be improved. Invite someone else to be the fieldworker and try a different approach.

Ask the group to take up roles of different members of a district health committee. One person acts as the health educator and tries to convince the others to work together to support a health education programme in the community. Problems of implementing health education programmes and overcoming bureaucratic resistance can be explored in the discussion afterwards.

Ask two people to act out a counselling situation with the others watching and afterwards discuss how successful it was. Another way of starting this is to use role cards (Figure 4.5) where situations are written down and a person has to pick one and the other has to respond. In the discussion afterwards, people can list the good points of communication and the bad points and thus find out for themselves the principles of successful face-to-face communication.

In role-play students can practise giving advice and making difficult decisions in a realistic situation. However, it is a 'safe' environment. You can make mistakes and try again, which is not possible in real life, where mistakes could have disastrous consequences. It is possible to try several versions of the answer and the group can discuss which role-play it thinks best and why. Role-plays can help a group:

- to get to know one another better;
- to think about a particular topic, problem or issue;
- to practise for a particular event such as a meeting or interview;
- to be more sympathetic to points of view of other people;
- to acquire social skills such as cooperation;
- to acquire communication or counselling skills.

Fig. 4.5 Example of a role card

The field worker has to give advice to the person showing the card and thus learns to understand how a woman feels when faced with additional demands from hygiene education programmes.

Problem-solving exercises, case studies and simulations

The best way to develop skills in problem-solving is to provide exercises where participants have to analyze a situation and decide on possible solutions. The problem can be in a real community or local clinic that the participants can visit and observe. You can then set a task which could be to:

- Design a leaflet about diarrhoea for mothers of under-fives.
- Suggest ways in which the health centre could improve its health education.
- Identify obstacles to promoting condoms; suggest how to overcome the difficulties.
- Suggest how schools and primary health services could work better together.
- Make a work-plan for reaching out-of-school children and prepare an action plan.

Field visits can take up a lot of time and transport may not be available. It is often more convenient to use *case studies* in which the problem is presented to the students in the form of a written report describing a situation. Case studies can be long or short, complex or simple, depending on the needs of the participants, the nature of the subject matter and the time available. The case study can be designed to reveal problems such as the failure of a health education programme. You can base it on fact or a pretended situation, but it should be as realistic as possible. Enough background information should be included, as well as questions setting out the tasks for the participants.

Participants can work on the problem in groups of 4–8 persons. You can allow as little as one hour or, with more complex problems, half a day or more. Groups can present their conclusions to the other participants verbally or as a written report.

Case studies can be combined with other methods. For example, you might use the case study as the basis for a role-play. *Simulations* are case studies where the participants each take on particular roles. For example you might assign each member of a group the role of a person in a district health team so they tackle the problem 'in role'.

Games

You can present information and ideas on health in exciting and challenging ways through games. Games are entertaining, they encourage cooperation and discussion and are good 'ice-breakers' at the beginning of a workshop to introduce participants and encourage an open approach to discussion. Some examples of games used in teaching about health include:

'Snakes and Ladders' where the snakes represent the causes of diarrhoea and the ladders are actions to prevent it.

Card games, e.g. a set of cards each containing a different activity, that the participants have to sort out into low, medium and high risk for transmission of HIV virus.

'Chinese whispers' – one person whispers a phrase to another who has to whisper it to the next person until it has passed through everyone. The final version is usually quite different from the original and in the discussion points are made about the distortion of messages that can occur through person-to-person communication in a community.

There are no fixed rules about how to go about developing a game. Start by deciding what knowledge and skills you want participants to learn. Use your imagination to think of interesting and different ways of communicating the points. Are there local games in your community that could be adapted?

Fig. 4.6 Learning aids for teaching about health

Using learning aids to improve your teaching

Learning aids can greatly improve your teaching – but only if they are well-chosen and properly used. A learning aid is only an *aid* to learning. Just showing a film, picture or slide by itself will only have a limited effect. Rather than using them just for formal one-way teaching they should be used to stimulate understanding, discussion and participatory learning.

Learning aids can
- keep the group's interest, arouse curiosity and hold attention;
- emphasise key points – when key headings are written out;
- allow step-by step explanation and sequencing of information;
- show something rather than just telling people – e.g. a jar of mosquito larvae, samples of condoms, drawing of a life-cycle of a disease; and
- provide a shared experience for discussion and questions.

An appropriate learning aid is:
- relevant to the learning objectives;
- affordable;
- easy to make and use;
- well understood by the audience;
- interesting and entertaining.
- It also encourages participation and discussion.

Demonstrations with real objects and models

In Chapter 2 you saw how people were more likely to believe something if they can see, feel, touch and smell it for themselves. It's always best to introduce real objects as learning aids. You could set up a display of food, make a field visit to inspect a latrine, pass out condoms for people to inspect and blow them into balloons to show how strong they are. However, it is often more convenient to use models rather than real objects. For example, models can be used to show a fruit which is out of season, a doll can be used to practise weighing or show the position of a baby during birth.

Using pictures in health education

Pictures can be useful learning aids if well-chosen and properly used. Many kinds of *visual aids* use pictures.

- A picture put up on a wall is called a *wallchart*. Because the teacher is there to explain, wallcharts can contain more information than a poster that has to be understood on its own.
- A *flashcard* is a picture shown to a group of people; it can be a single picture but more often a series of pictures.
- It is easy to drop a set of flash cards by accident and mix them up. A *flip chart* is a series of pictures that are attached together – usually with a spiral binding so they can be turned over one at a time.
- Other ways of using pictures include *flannelgraphs, slides and overhead projector transparencies*.

In the previous chapter you saw how easy it can be for people to misunderstand pictures. Wherever possible try to use the real thing or models – do not show a picture of a condom when you can show a real one. If it is not possible to show the real thing, a model might be easier to understand than a picture. If you decide to use pictures, pre-test them with a sample of your intended audience and make certain that they can be understood.

How pictures can be used to promote learning

Well-chosen and properly used pictures can:
1. Convey visual information, e.g. what a latrine looks like.
2. Show something people cannot see in real life, e.g. internal structure of genital organs.
3. Provide a substitute for the real thing if it is difficult to obtain e.g. pictures of out-of-season foods, or a picture of child with particular symptoms.
4. Make difficult ideas easier to understand (*showing rather than telling*), e.g. making something small look larger, comparisons of similarities and differences, showing how something changes or grows, showing steps in doing a task.
5. Help people remember key points.
6. Arouse people's interest and gain attention.
7. Act as a stimulus for participatory learning and development of problem-solving skills, e.g. picture posing a problem for which the group is invited to offer solutions, a sequence of pictures that the group is asked to put in an order that makes sense to them.

Flannelgraphs

Flannelgraphs are pictures with a rough back which allows the picture to stick to a cloth. The picture can be printed on cloth or paper with a rough backing such as sandpaper. The board can be a blanket or cloth stuck to a board. Flannelgraphs have several advantages as visual aids:

- They are easily carried by a field worker without a vehicle. They do not need electricity or expensive equipment to use.
- If they are properly stored, the pictures can be used repeatedly.

Fig. 4.7 The flannelgraph

- They are simple and clear. They provide a visual framework on which to hang ideas.
- The subject can be built up picture by picture. Negative ideas can be replaced by positive ones and the scene can move and change.
- The pictures can be left up for as long as necessary for questions and discussion.
- They are quick to set up and use, in homes or in a group.
- They can be added to and adapted by the people using them.
- Flannelgraphs are easily used to encourage audience participation.

Slides

Slides or transparencies are photographs taken with 35 mm colour 'reversal' film that can be projected on a screen or white wall. Slides can be used to project colour photographs to a large size so a group of 20 or more people can see them. The organization Teaching Aids at Low Cost makes available slide sets on a wide range of health topics (see Appendix C).

Slides can be used in many ways. You can encourage learner-participation by inviting your audience to discuss what they see in the slide. Even better, you can ask them to come forward and point out key topics.

You do not have to use all the slides in a set but can select the ones that are relevant to your need. This is especially useful if the slides have been produced in another country. Any 35 mm camera can be used to take slides. So it is easy to take photographs locally either to make up a complete set or to include in one that you have bought.

Films and videos

The 16 mm film projector has been widely used in educational work. However, video is increasingly becoming affordable. Both have the advantage over 'still' photographs of showing movement and actions. This is particularly useful if you want to show skills such as building a latrine or organizing a drama session. They are also very good for attracting an audience and keeping their attention. However, one problem with films is that they need a blackout. Video does not need a darkened room, but the size of the screen is too small to use with a large group. If your audience is not familiar with film or video, there is a danger that they may see them as sources of entertainment rather than for instruction and learning. Never rely entirely on the film or video to convey the message. Always introduce the film beforehand to point out any special feature and afterwards summarize and discuss with the group the key points to make sure that they have been understood. Some suggestions for using films and videos are given in the list.

Video programmes are easier to produce than film and you could try to find out if there are production facilities near you. You could even try to work with film-makers to produce your own! Sometimes useful programmes are broadcast on television and you can get permission to videotape them for use in your educational work.

Using films and videos

Questions to ask when choosing the film or video
1. Is the technical quality good – i.e. sound and picture quality?
2. What audience is it suitable for – children, the general public, health workers, student health workers, others?

3. Is it interesting?
4. Is it culturally acceptable to your audience and unlikely to cause offence?
5. Is it relevant and appropriate to your problems and your ways of dealing with them?
6. Is the health content accurate?
7. Can it be used to stimulate discussion?

Before showing it

Go early and set everything up, check that all equipment is working and the film or video is not damaged. Give a short introduction to the audience.

Give them hints about what to look for.

Explain words which they may find difficult.

Warn them about any parts of the film or video that you feel are not correct, or might distract them from the teaching points of the film.

Make sure everyone has a clear view of the screen.

During the showing

Stay near the projector or video recorder in case there are serious problems or to adjust, the sound, focus, etc.

After it is finished

Discuss the film with the audience. This lets you see whether they have observed the teaching points and explain any confusions.

The overhead projector

The overhead projector is becoming increasingly popular as a learning aid. It provides a bright picture in daylight so does not need a darkened room. When using it, you face the audience and do not have to turn your back to them. It is cheap to buy, simple to use and maintain. You can prepare transparencies in advance and when you finish your teaching, they can be stored for the next time you need them. Unfortunately many people do not use the overhead projector to its best advantage and the words are too small, crowded and not clear. The guidelines in the list describe a range of imaginative and active ways of using the overhead projector and designing effective transparencies.

Hints on using the overhead projector

MAKING THE TRANSPARENCIES

1. DESIGN your transparencies carefully. Plan them before you put pen to acetate.
2. KEEP IT SIMPLE – present one main idea on each sheet.
   Aim for not more than 10 lines of lettering per transparency and maximum of seven words a line.
   Use different colours to emphasize points (but do not use too many).
3. Always check that the words can be read from the back of the room. If you do copy diagrams make sure that they are large enough as most diagrams and words in books are too small. You might be able to obtain access to a photocopier which can enlarge pictures. Typewriting is too small, lettering should be at least 6 mm. Use lower case letters wherever possible as they are easier to read.
4. Try whenever possible to replace words with pictures. If you are not very good at drawing look out for pictures in books. It is easy to place a transparency over them to copy.
5. Use a piece of lined paper under the acetate to keep your writing straight.
6. Margin – the edge of an overhead transparency is often not projected so leave

How it works

COMPONENT PARTS

Despite the diversity of overhead projector designs, the basic elements of their optical systems are the same: —

1. a powerful light source, usually a small Tungsten-Halogen bulb;
2. some kind of reflector behind it to concentrate the light;
3. a condensing system (usually containing a Fresnel lens — a convex plastic lens with moulded concentric wedge-form rings) to direct light through the transparency stage on to the objective lens;
4. a transparency stage or platen;
5. an objective lens to focus the projected image on to a screen;
6. a plane mirror to change the direction of the light rays (the objective lens often comprises two lenses with the mirror between them).

This optical system is usually arranged so that the projector looks something like this:

Fig. 4.8 The overhead projector

84

the overhead projector

2 cm round the edge. It is a good idea to draw a border around the transparency as it focuses attention on the content.

7. Use overhead projector pens. Pens with water-based ink have the advantage of being easily erased with a damp cloth and the transparency can be reused. However, in hot humid conditions they easily smudge. 'Permanent' pens have a spirit-based ink. You can erase them within the first few minutes of use with methylated spirits but once they have dried they are difficult to remove and the transparency cannot be reused.

8. Acetate sheets for overhead transparencies come in different thicknesses – thicker ones last longer but are more expensive. Many photocopiers can copy diagrams on to special acetate sheets – check the instructions!

SHOWING THE TRANSPARENCIES

1. Position yourself, the projector and screen carefully – make sure the audience's view of the screen is not blocked – and face the audience.

2. Switch off between transparencies – switching on the OHP is a signal and brings people's attention back to the screen.

3. Leave each transparency up long enough for the audience to absorb the information. Avoid the temptation to rush to the next visual.

4. Point out details on the transparency itself, not on the screen. You can use a pen as a pointer.

5. Some of the different ways of using an overhead transparency include:
   transparency rolls – writing points down as you go on rolls of acetate.
   'reveal method' – covering the transparency with a sheet of paper that is lowered step-by-step to reveal the words or pictures as you talk about them.
   masking – masking off areas and revealing them in turn as appropriate.
   overlays – one sheet of acetate laid over another to build up information and more detail.

Putting it all together – planning a lesson

You should now be in a position to apply the ideas presented above to planning your teaching.

ADVANCE PREPARATION AND PLANNING

1. Prepare the talk, finding out the needs and background knowledge of the target group and size of group.
2. Write out objectives of the topic you want to put over.
3. Decide how much is to be covered in one session and ask:
   What sequence should the information be presented in to make it as logical as possible?
   What questions can I ask to check that the information is understood?
   If skills are to be taught, how can I demonstrate the skill to the group? What opportunities can be provided to practise the skills either in the class or a real-life setting?
   How can you best share the ideas you want to put across?
   By having a discussion, demonstration, telling a story, acting out a drama?
   By showing some pictures, playing a game?
4. Write an outline of your main points. (Avoid writing out the whole lecture, otherwise you will just read it out and sound boring.)
5. Prepare and practise using the visual aids you think will help in getting the information across.
   Can key points and ideas be shown in pictures?
   What learning aids can I use to explain these facts more clearly?
   Can I put the most important information on a hand-out?
6. Check all the equipment, e.g. overhead projector, slide projector, extension cords, spare bulbs, etc. that you need are available and in good working order and the room is set up before the participants arrive.

RUNNING THE TEACHING SESSION

- Introduce yourself and the topic – get everyone's attention.
- Give a summary of the main points you will cover.
- Present your facts and information showing relevant visual aids when appropriate.
- Speak loud and clear so everyone can hear.
- Make sure your language is suited to your audience.
- Try not to be distracting by too much moving around or mannerisms, e.g. jangling keys.
- Keep a constant watch on the reactions of the group to your teaching. Look out for signs of misunderstanding or boredom in the class. Actively encourage questions.
- Provide practical assignments or reading to follow on from the lecture. Handouts listing the main points are often useful. Evaluate the session by asking questions or setting a task.

Organizing training programmes and workshops

Bringing people together is a costly process in travel, food and disrupted work schedules. Face-to-face teaching sessions should be kept to a minimum. Concentrate on activities that *cannot* be learnt through distance learning such as attitudes, decision-making, communication and psycho-motor skills. Can any of your objectives be achieved through distance learning methods? These could be newsletters, talks on the radio or audio-cassettes and handbooks. The correspondence course is one form of distance education where reading materials, cassettes and even slides are sent to fieldworkers with exercises and field activities. Feedback

Fig. 4.9 Decision-making for planning training

is given to the fieldworkers by post. Local fieldworkers can be given training to enable them to act as field supervisors.

Once you have decided that a training workshop is needed you need to plan it properly. One of the biggest problems in training is ensuring that what has been learnt is actually applied in real life. Careful attention to the selection of participants, timing, place of training, content, teaching methods and follow-up will help to make sure that your training activities will be put into practice.

Selection of participants

You will have to consider carefully how you will make sure that you get the course-participants you want. The ideal situation is to have participants who are of the right educational level and experience to benefit from the course, who are enthusiastic and motivated and can put into practice their newly-learnt ideas and skills. If you are running a community-based programme, the participants will probably have been chosen by the community themselves. It is important to get a good 'mix' of participants, especially male and female workers, background disciplines and experiences. Unfortunately, people may be sent to a training workshop for a variety of reasons – because of seniority, because it is their turn to have a 'day off' or personal connections.

Choice of place for training

Good teaching rooms, food and accommodation facilities are important; also, a training course will be more likely to be put into practice if it is carried out in a realistic field-setting where relevant field exercises can be included in the training.

87

Some people criticize the approach of bringing participants together to a training centre. An alternative is to run the training in the field centre with all the fieldworkers in the local team joining in. This way they can discuss how they can put it into practice in their situation. However it is often a good idea to give people a chance to leave the pressures of their work to reflect on what they have been doing. A useful approach is to take two or three people from a single work-setting. After the course they can continue to discuss what they have learnt and can support each other in putting the ideas into practice.

Timing the sessions

Carrying out all the teaching in one continuous course is not always the best approach. One way to encourage putting into practice is to split the training course into two or more blocks of teaching with gaps in between. You can ask the participants to carry out reading and practical exercises in their workplace during the interval before their next course. When they come back together as a group you can then discuss the problems of putting the new ideas they have learnt into their practice. For example, if you have five days available for training you could use them in different ways as shown in Figure 4.10.

'day release' one day per session	x	x	x	x	x
3-day course with two follow-up days	xxx		x		x
3-day course with 2-day follow-up course	xxx		xx		

x = one day's training

Fig. 4.10 Different ways of using five days' training

Organization of the content

At the beginning of any training there should be a session to find out the background experiences of the participants and what they feel they need to know. This also helps to 'break the ice' and start the participants talking and getting to know each other. You can then introduce the aims of the training which you can change to take into account their interests. They are much more likely to pay attention and learn from their training if they have participated in discussions about the content and felt needs are met. You could even send out a questionnaire to all participants before the course begins to find out their views.

Keep the timetable flexible so that you can include any additional topics that arise and the participants want to discuss further. Include review sessions where you look back at what has been covered and look ahead at the next part of the programme. It is a good idea to ask the participants to select representatives who can discuss any special needs and problems. Avoid the temptation to put too much into a timetable. People need the opportunity to relax in the evenings and at meals otherwise they will get tired and lose concentration.

A good way of encouraging participants to put into practice their training is to provide a 'where do we go from here?' session at the end. They can prepare action plans for putting the new ideas into practice in their workplace and can present these plans to the other participants. You can follow this up with a discussion of possible obstacles to implementing their plans and how these obstacles can be overcome.

One problem with training courses is that they are taught as series of separate topics, e.g. how to do a community profile, advantages of community participation, use of educational methods. At the end of the course, participants find it difficult to put it all into practice. An alternative to the traditional subject-based approach is a problem-solving approach to the teaching. This approach begins with a problem, e.g. how do we improve weaning practices in the community? How can latrines be promoted? How can we get young people to practise safe sex? Participants then carry out a series of activities in field situations to solve the problem. At various points in the course, trainers introduce key ideas. Participants will then be in a better position to apply the ideas gained in the course.

In one of my training courses at Leeds, I asked a group of students from Africa, Asia and the Caribbean to write down all the bad things they had experienced in workshops and all the good ones as well. The list of bad points was very long. Although workshops are widely used for introducing new ideas to fieldworkers, they are often not done very well. Typical problems are: overloaded and irrelevant content; poor facilities; inappropriate and overcrowded timetable; over-use of formal lectures and not enough discussion/practical activities; failure to consult the participants; poor organization. It is not surprising that people do not put the ideas from workshops into practice! We followed up our discussions of good and bad points by preparing the checklist for planning an effective workshop shown in the list just before the Summary at the end of this chapter.

Evaluation of training programmes

You will need to give some thought to how you will *evaluate* your workshop and some possible evaluation questions are listed here. Training programmes are evaluated for many different reasons: in the short term you will want to make sure that participants have mastered the tasks and learning components in the course; in the long term you will need to find out if they are actually putting into practice the new ideas they have learnt and if they are having an impact on the health of the community.

Questions to ask when evaluating a training programme

Short-term evaluation
Were the participants satisfied with the content of the course?
Were there topics that they would have liked to have seen included?
Was it taught in an interesting way?
Were the food, accommodation and social arrangements satisfactory?
At the end of the course were they able to perform to a satisfactory level the skills identified in the task analysis and course objective?
Do the participants feel confident that they can put into practice their new skills?
Is there a need for follow-up training?
Are there any general recommendations on policy from the participants?
Long-term evaluation
Are the participants satisfied with their training?
Do they have any further suggestions on training content?
Are the participants putting into practice what they have learnt?
What obstacles, if any, are preventing them from undertaking their tasks?
Are their employers satisfied with the results of the training?

Are the community satisfied with the results of the training?
What impact have their activities had upon the health of the community?
Is there a need for follow-up training?

Guidelines on running workshops

Before the workshop
- Form an organizing committee to plan the workshop with clearly-defined responsibilities for each member.
- Have clearly-defined objectives for the workshop; specify date and length of the workshop.
- Decide who the participants will be and how many should come; visit participants, where possible in their workplace, to discuss the workshop and ask for suggestions on content. Where a personal visit is not possible, send a questionnaire to participants in which they can identify their needs; send out invitations to participants well in advance; check that they can come and have a reserve list if people drop out.
- Identify external speakers and chairpersons for sessions; have meetings with resource persons and facilitators to brief them and identify any required resources; identify a person to open and close the workshop; give everybody plenty of notice; check they can come.
- Choose the place where the workshop is taking place including the accommodation, teaching rooms; inspect and check lighting, size, seating, recreational facilities during the evening, toilet facilities; speak to the local administrator of the facility (and the catering officer if a separate person) and explain requirements; confirm the booking.
- Plan the timetable; prepare a social programme with some visits and evening activities.
- Arrange for typing and duplicating facilities during the workshop.
- Make a budget providing for transport, hire of rooms, food, accommodation, materials, speaker's expenses, hire of equipment, secretarial expenses; submit the budget to the finance office, ensure approval and that money is available.
- Order required materials, stationery, pens, paper; arrange for printing of handouts and timetable; obtain any learning aids required including flipcharts, videos, etc. Invite media to the opening and the close of the workshop and send out a press release.

During the workshop
- Register participants; issue name badges, timetables, notepads; organize financial arrangements.
- Brief participants (introduction and 'icebreaking').
- Give out a pre-test questionnaire of participants (if one has not been given before); discuss the participants' expectations.
- Form a workshop committee with involvement of participants.
- Make yourself available to sort out problems as and when they occur.
- Obtain feedback at the end of the day; get proceedings of each day typed up, monitoring the timetable where necessary.
- Keep a written record of any recommendations and resolutions.
- Evaluate at the end of the workshop.

After the workshop
- Return all borrowed equipment and materials.
- Prepare report with the workshop recommendations and send it to decision-makers, sponsors and participants.

- Write to all resource persons and thank them for participation.
- Pay all outstanding bills and produce final budget.
- Hold meeting of organizing committee to discuss workshop report and follow-up.

Summary

This chapter has looked at some of the issues you should consider in planning effective programmes of teaching and training. The main points can be summarized as:

1. Decide on the overall objectives for the teaching; this is done by analysis of the tasks to be performed and involvement of the participants themselves.
2. Analyze the kinds of learning involved in carrying out the task; this involves identifying the need for learning facts, skills (decision-making, psycho-motor and communication) and attitudes.
3. Choose appropriate teaching methods for each type of learning; include active methods of learning, including problem-solving, role play and field exercises; select appropriate learning aids.
4. Prepare a plan for the training; decide on selection of participants, duration and timing of training, location of training, timetable for the programme, resources (equipment and staff), assessment of performance.
5. Carry out short-term and long-term evaluation of the teaching activity.

5. Face-to-face

This chapter will look at some of the ways in which you can work effectively with individuals and small groups. It will build on the discussions of communication and teaching methods in the previous two chapters and explore:

1. Different kinds of *one-to-one* communication ranging from simple instructions to problem-solving counselling and how these can be carried out.
2. The role of groups in health education and health promotion and methods for working in groups.
3. Ways in which the effectiveness of face-to-face communication can be improved.
4. Putting face-to-face communication into practice in patient education programmes.

In previous chapters many special advantages of face-to-face or 'person-to-person' communication were discussed. Face-to-face methods have a number of advantages over mass media such as radio or leaflets. It is possible to make the advice specific to the needs of your audience. You can find out how much they know already by asking questions at the beginning of a session and change the advice you are giving. You can also ask questions at the end of a session and discover how well understood and convincing you have been!

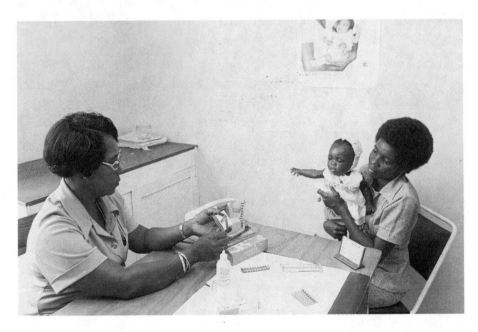

Fig. 5.1 Face-to-face communication has many advantages

Non-verbal communication

Face-to-face communication involves different kinds of communication. The most obvious communication takes place through the actual words – *verbal communication*. You will already have looked at communication difficulties from using complicated unfamiliar words in Chapter 3. Unfortunately some people deliberately use long technical words as a way of showing off and acting superior.

Much communication also takes place through *non-verbal communication* which was also introduced in Chapter 3. Table 5.1 summarizes the many different kinds of non-verbal communication that includes all those aspects of communication between people which do not involve the actual meaning of words. Most of us think a great deal about choosing the words we say when talking with another person. However, we often forget to plan our non-verbal communication. But the gestures we use, how we look at people, our tone of voice, how we are seated and our clothes can all have an impact on the way people interpret what we say.

We use non-verbal communication continually in everyday contact. For example, you might decide that a person is not telling the truth because he doesn't 'look' convincing. People express anger, love, sympathy and other emotions through their non-verbal communication. Points in conversations are emphasized through gestures and head-nodding. An important feedback on whether people are listening comes from nods, sounds of agreements, 'ums and ahs' and looks of encouragement (see Table 5.1). It is a useful exercise just to watch people talking and look out for non-verbal communication. You can also learn a great deal about non-verbal communication by turning down the sound when watching television or speeding up the motion on a videotape recorder.

In your face-to-face communication you have to be sensitive to the impact our non-verbal communication might be having. For example: sitting behind a desk can reinforce the barrier between health worker and community; looking at

Table 5.1 Different kinds of non-verbal communication

Sounds accompanying spoken words
pitch of voice
'um's, er's' and other sounds
laughing, angry, groaning
pauses
speed of talking
stresses on particular words
loudness or softness

Body language

body contact	touching, holding hands, caressing, greetings, shaking hands
closeness	distance between persons
posture	sitting up, slouching, leaning forward
orientation	angle at which people put themselves
gestures	hand movements, shaking and nodding head
gaze/looks	eye movements, raising eyebrows, shape of mouth
appearance	clothes, hair, cleanliness

---

your watch, looking away or writing down notes might be taken as showing boredom; and talking loudly may seem a sign of anger.

Non-verbal communication can be interpreted in different ways according to the culture of the community and this can also lead to misunderstandings. For example, in Western cultures much importance is given to looking people straight in the eye. In other cultures looking directly at someone in the face can be considered rude and showing lack of respect. Greetings and ways of showing sympathy can vary according to the culture.

So in your contacts with other people, either individually or in groups, you have to become sensitive to your own non-verbal communication. It is not enough to listen and feel sympathetic and concerned for the other persons. You have to be able to *show* it.

One-to-one

The one-to-one situation is very important in health education. Situations where one-to-one communication takes place include meetings between doctors and patients, home visits in the community and discussions with individuals in communities and can include:

simple giving of information;
persuading someone to undertake a particular action;
helping someone to take a decision, e.g. which contraceptive method to use;
breaking sensitive news, e.g. that the person is infected with HIV virus;
helping someone to cope with a difficult situation; and
therapy for someone who has a particular problem, e.g. is an alcoholic.

Counselling

In traditional advice-giving, the health worker is often trying to persuade a person to follow a particular course of action. Counselling is a process that goes beyond

Fig. 5.2 One-to-one communication

94

simply giving information but involves helping people *to make decisions* and giving them the confidence to put their decisions into practice. A difficulty we all have is to avoid imposing our own views on others. We need to try to understand our own values, opinions and prejudices so that we don't impose our own values on others. Counselling is based on the following assumptions:

- Counselling should take into account psycho-social, financial and spiritual needs of the client.
- Everything said during a counselling session should be treated as strictly confidential.
- Any information provided should be clearly put, accurate and consistent.
- The emphasis should be that of promoting informed decision-making; the counsellor avoids giving direct advice but instead helps the person to make decisions for himself or herself.
- The client has the right to choose his or her own actions.

Eight common reasons for breakdown of one-to-one communication

---

1. The communication is carried out in a place where there is a lot of noise and distractions.
2. The person feels uncomfortable and distracted, is too self-conscious to discuss problems because of people overhearing or does not really trust the health educator.
3. The health educator does not find out the real reasons for the problem, uses complicated language with unfamiliar terms, gives advice that is irrelevant or impossible to put into practice.
4. People go away with doubts and questions they felt they could not raise with the health worker.
5. Most people want to be told more about their illnesses than the doctor is willing to say.
6. Too much information is given; the person only remembers part of what was said during the meeting – especially if he/she is anxious and worried.
7. There is a wide difference in background between the two persons without enough sharing of culture, perceptions, beliefs and values to allow communication and understanding. Insufficient time is available to find out what the person's problems really are or properly explain the facts.
8. There is no follow-up to check if the advice is put into practice.

Promoting effective one-to-one communication

Many studies have been carried out on communication between health workers and their patients to find out the reasons why patients do not follow the advice given. Some of the problems that these studies have identified are shown in the list and in Figure 5.3.

For effective one-to-one communication three sets of factors are important: the place and time when the communication takes place; the handling of the actual encounter; and obtaining feedback on its effectiveness.

The place and time

If you are seeing people at a health centre, you should try to set aside a place

Fig. 5.3 Blocks to communication. What difference do you see between the two situations in the illustration?

where you can talk to them in private without interruptions. If you do not have much time to spare, or have others to see as well, you can ask the person to return later when you have more free time. If you have a receptionist to answer the telephone, ask for any calls to be intercepted during the session.

Handling the encounter

The way you conduct your session – talking and listening – will have an impact on its effectiveness. You may find the GATHER approach described opposite a useful checklist as well as the guidelines below:

- Put the person at ease at the beginning of the session with a smile and a greeting.
- Choose carefully what advice to give so that it is relevant, and realistic; be selective about the amount of information you give in any one session. The more information you provide the more likely it will be that the person will forget what you are saying – aim to make three or four key points.
- Make your advice as specific as possible – instead of saying 'practise good hygiene', say 'Wash your hands before preparing your baby's food.'
- Use simple language – avoid technical terms.
- Give information in an organized way: 'I am going to tell you three things you can do. The first is . . . the second is . . . and the third is . . .'
- Give the most important advice first and repeat it at the end .
- Check that your main points have been understood, by asking questions such as 'Now please explain back to me how often you should take the pills.'
- Provide a leaflet with the key points for the person to take away.

We often are so concerned with giving advice that we do not listen to what people themselves want to know. *Listening* is an important part of handling the encounter. Some common problems in listening include the following:

- **daydreaming** – because we can think faster than people can talk to us we can easily become distracted and think of other things and miss important points;

96

- *jumping to conclusions* – we jump to conclusions about what people are going to say so we do not really pay attention;
- *reacting to specific words* – we react strongly to certain words such as money, lack of time, family problems and stop listening;
- *turning off* when the subject is complicated – if the topic is complicated and involved we can turn off and stop listening.

When you are listening to someone, try to avoid: passing judgement either in words or through your looks and gestures; arguing; interrupting and rushing them; and jumping to conclusions. Listening is an *active* process. You should continually show interest and provide encouragement and pay attention by looking at the person. Try to give the person time to explain their situation. Do not be afraid to allow moments of silence while they are collecting their thoughts. You should ask for clarification on any points you do not understand.

Obtaining feedback on the outcome of the session

This is the third ingredient for effective one-to-one communication. This can be asking questions. For example, you could ask what the person intends to do and whether he or she feels that they can put into practice the advice you have given. You will have to ask in a sensitive way; you might be told what they think you want to hear rather than what they really believe. You could ask the person to return at a future date when you can look for improvements in health. You could also make a follow-up visit to the person's home or ask someone else to pay a visit and observe them.

The GATHER approach to one-to-one communication

G   **Greet the person**: put them at ease, show respect and trust; emphasize the confidential nature of the discussion.

A   **Ask about their problem**: encourage them to bring out their anxieties, worries and needs, determine their access to support and help in their family and community; find out what steps they have already taken to deal with the situation; encourage the person to express their feelings in their own words; show respect and tolerance to what they say and do not pass judgement; actively listen and show that you are paying attention through your looking; encourage them through helpful questions.

T   **Tell them any relevant information** they need: provide accurate and specific information in reply to their questions; give information on what they can do to help their health, explain any background information they need to know about the particular health issue; keep your language simple, repeat important points and ask questions to check that the important points are understood; provide the important information in the form of a leaflet that they can take away.

H   **Help them to make decisions**: explore the various alternatives; raise issues they may not have thought of; be careful of letting your own views, values and prejudices influence the advice you give; ensure that it is their own decision and not one that you have imposed; help them make a plan of action.

E   **Explain any misunderstandings**: ask questions to check understanding of important points; ask the person to repeat back in their own words the key points.

R   **Return to follow up on them**: make arrangements for a follow-up visit or referral to other agencies; if a follow-up visit is not necessary, give the name of someone they can contact it they need help.

Working with groups

There are many different reasons why we work in groups for our health education and health promotion work.

Problem-solving groups and teams

Planning and implementing your educational activities will usually involve setting up groups such as committees or working in teams with other people. You may need to set up groups in order to: solve problems and make decisions, bring together a set of skills, talents and responsibilities to find the best possible solution to a problem; collect information and ideas; gather ideas, information or make suggestions; and coordinate and liaise the activities of different persons.

Teaching/learning groups

You will have seen in the previous chapter that teaching with small groups has many advantages. You can use groups to: develop problem-solving skills; encourage learner participation, discussion and feedback; explore values and beliefs; and deal with sensitive issues such as sex.

Community-based groups

Community participation programmes usually set up committees to manage the programme, make decisions and liaise with the health services (see Chapter 6). The success or failure of community participation programmes will depend heavily on how well these groups function and on how much support they receive.

Self-help groups

Belonging to a small group can benefit members directly through the help they can give each other. Support and practical advice from someone else who has had a similar problem is often more useful than receiving advice from a health worker. Many people with problems can feel very isolated and find it helpful to meet others with similar experiences. Self-help groups have been set up on many different topics and some examples are given here.

Fig. 5.4 Group discussion

98

Examples of self-help groups

Alcoholics Anonymous where all the members are alcoholics and help each other to stop drinking.

Breastfeeding support groups where women who are breastfeeding meet, share experiences, help each other and receive help from other women who have successfully breastfed.

AIDS support groups, e.g. 'Body positive' – groups of persons who are HIV antibody positive regularly meet to provide each other support and encouragement.

Colostomy support groups – people who have had a colostomy operation involving removal of part of their colon so that their faeces emerge from an opening on their side into a plastic bag. This support group involves meeting and sharing experiences, discuss coping strategies, briefing people who are about to have the operation.

Stop smoking groups – people who want to give up smoking form a group and regularly meet to provide support and monitor each other's progress.

The different kinds of groups listed overlap. You might set up a group within a community-based programme and then undertake some small-group teaching activity with it. You may hold a group teaching session with patients at a clinic, e.g. leprosy patients, and encourage them to continue as a self-help group to provide each other with mutual support. You might form a liaison committee to run a health education programme in your district and conduct a small-group teaching session to introduce a new skill.

Problems in group functioning

Working in groups can be highly effective and get good results. It can also be frustrating, difficult and lead to failures. Think about your own experiences with groups – what problems have you encountered? Have any of your own experiences of difficulties included any of the following?

Lack of a common purpose; everyone wants something different.

Some individuals dominate the discussion, others are silent and do not contribute.

Disagreements, personality clashes and conflicts among the members.

Members fail to perform assigned tasks.

Poor and irregular attendance.

Everyone talks but nobody is willing to make decisions.

Fig. 5.5 Meetings

Group dynamics

The functioning of groups has been called *group dynamics*. Social psychologists have studied group dynamics and have found the following to be very important in determining the effectiveness of group functioning: the characteristics of the group including size and membership; the nature of the tasks undertaken; the decision-making processes; the roles of members; group processes; and pattern of leadership.

Characteristics of the group

Here are some definitions of what constitutes a group:

'a group is best defined as a dynamic whole based on interdependence rather than similarity' (*Lewin*)

'the distinctive thing about a group is that its members share norms about something' (*Newcomb*)

'engaged in interaction with one another in a single face-to-face meeting or series of such meetings' (*Bales*)

A group is not just a collection of people – they should *share some characteristics and interact*. Because of this interaction, a group is more than the sum of the individuals that make it up. The group acquires its own characteristics.

Size of group

A group can have as few as four people and as many as 24. The kinds of interactions, opportunities for exchange of ideas and success in achieving objectives are affected by the group size. With too few members most people will have a chance to contribute, but there will be less experience to draw on from the members. With too many people, it is difficult for everyone to contribute in discussion and it will be harder to reach a shared decision. Many feel that 8–12 persons is an ideal size for a group but it really depends on the aims and purpose of the group.

Background of the group members

Who the group members are and their reasons for attending are of enormous importance. If the members have been sent by their employers to attend, they may not really be interested in the group – they may even feel that their selection is a punishment. Persons may have a 'hidden agenda' and see the function of the group as meeting their own personal or employer's wishes. Other ways in which individual behaviours help or hinder the group are described below in the section on group processes. You may have no choice but to accept into the group whoever has been sent. However, wherever possible, try to involve people who you know will work well with others.

The nature of the task

Some of the different kinds of tasks that groups are concerned with were described at the beginning of this section. Another way of thinking about different kinds of groups is the extent to which they are mainly concerned with producing results (task-oriented) or with promoting the well-being of the members of the groups (process-oriented) – see Figure 5.6.

Group decision-making

Every group is constantly making decisions. Some decisions may be small, others may be large ones with important consequences. How well those decisions are

TASK-ORIENTED
(directed outwards to achieve tasks)

a) "mini lecture"
b) seminar
c) syndicate/enquiry-based group
d) committees
e) brainstorming groups
f) community-based group
g) value clarification group
h) developmental group
i) group discussion–decision
j) 'T' (sensitivity) group
k) encounter group
l) therapy or self-help group

PROCESS-ORIENTED
(inwards-looking for benefit of members)

Fig. 5.6 Process and task-oriented groups

made will depend on many factors, including: complexity of the decision required; the range of skills/expertise in the group and the amount of relevant information available to the members. One way of reaching a decision in a group is through *consensus* – with everyone's agreement. This is often the best way – provided you are sure that everyone really does agree and is not just keeping silent because they feel inhibited to give their opinion. With a larger group it can be difficult to get everyone to agree. A vote can be taken and the majority view followed. But if you do make decisions by voting, you must take care that those with minority views do not feel left out and drop out of future activities.

Some of the different reasons why groups find it difficult to make decisions are given here. To overcome these problems, the group must be honest with itself and openly discuss them and try to find a solution. Good leadership is essential to resolve these difficulties and make effective decisions.

Obstacles to group decision-making

fear of consequences: fear that employers or other influential people will criticize them for taking a particular decision.
conflicting loyalties: there can be divided loyalties among the different members to employers, communities, churches etc.
disagreements and personalities: personal behaviour and disagreements between group members can interfere with decision-making (see section on individual behaviour).
hidden agenda: individual group members may try to influence the whole group to follow their particular interests.
inadequate information: the decision may be based on the personal opinions of the group members rather than the facts of the situation.

During a group's activities, members can take a range of roles – some helpful and others unhelpful. A workshop held in Zambia by the Economic Commission for Africa identified the following characteristics and provided hints on how to deal with them.

The quarrelsome type. Keep cool. Don't allow yourself to become involved in an argument. Ask them questions and they will probably make some foolish or far-fetched statements that can be dealt with by other group members. Don't allow anyone to become personal.

The positive type. They can be of great help to the chairperson, particularly when the discussion gets bogged down. Use them frequently but don't let them monopolize the conversation.

The know-all type. They may be bluffing and not really know the answers. When they give an opinion ask them to give reasons. If the reasons seem faulty ask other members of the group to comment. This helps to build up confidence in the group so they will not be imposed on.

The talkative type. Don't discourage them. If they are well-informed their opinion can be of help to the group. If they talk for too long they can bore others. Be prepared to interrupt them tactfully and ask a direct question of someone else.

The shy type. They may know a great deal but be shy to speak out. Often the talkative and know-all types are the men; the women may be more shy but have much of importance to contribute to the group. When suitable opportunities arise, call upon them by name to give an opinion but be sure that the question is an easy one to build up confidence to contribute more to the group.

The uncooperative rejecting type. Be patient and try to win their friendship. Acknowledge their experience and let them feel that you depend upon their help for the success of the meeting.

The highbrow intellectual type. Be patient, but keep to the point; if necessary, rephrase their statements for the benefit of other members. Ask them to help the group with difficult technical points. Take care that they do not over-awe the rest of the group and make them feel inadequate.

The persistent questioner. They are often out to trap the chairperson. Pass their questions back to the group and then get the questioner's views.

Some other kinds of difficult group behaviour were identified in that same workshop and given the personalities of animals!

The **donkey** – who is very stubborn and will not change his point of view 'I will not be moved'.

The **lion** – who fights whenever others disagree with his plans or interfere with his desires.

The **rabbit** – who runs away when he senses tension or conflict or switches quickly to another topic.

The **ostrich** – who buries his head in the sand and refuses to admit any problem at all.

The **monkey** – who fools around and prevents the group from concentrating on serious business.

The **hyena** – who laughs and makes jokes to avoid dealing with difficulties or puts rivals down.

The **elephant** – who blocks the way and stubbornly prevents the group from continuing along the road to their desired goals.

The *giraffe* – who looks down on others and on the programme in general, feeling that 'I am above it all'.

The *tortoise* – who withdraws from the group, refusing to give ideas or opinions.

The *cat* – who is always looking for sympathy. 'It is so difficult for me.'

The *peacock* – who is always competing for attention. 'See what a fine fellow I am.'

Stages in setting up a group

One useful approach shown in Table 5.2 is to separate out the various stages of establishing a group: the setting-up stage or 'forming'; the action stage or 'storming'; and the establishing stage or 'norming'. Some of the issues you should consider at each stage are shown in Table 5.2 and you will probably notice some similarities with the stages in community participation described in Chapter 6.

Table 5.2 Stages in group formation and action

SETTING UP ▼	create climate of trust between members
	share expectations
	understand each person's personal objectives
	agree on objectives for group
	review membership and involve others if needed
	agree on strategy for achieving objectives
ACTION ▼	obtain necessary data
	set up working groups
	make decisions
	implement activities
ESTABLISHING	evaluate activities
	reflect on achievements
	review objectives
	make future plans
	review membership and involve others
	if necessary, decide to end group

In the setting-up stage it is essential to create a climate of trust. Everyone should feel free to give their opinion, share ideas and be prepared to work together to achieve the objectives. You have to look out for people who have hidden reasons for attending. Others may have come only because they have been told to attend by their employers but are really not very interested. Have you left out anyone important from the membership?

The action stage depends a great deal on the quality of leadership, which is discussed below. Only a limited range of topics can be handled in detail by a group at any one meeting. Large meetings are good for obtaining agreement on broad points. However, they can be inefficient for detailed work such as preparing a curriculum, writing a leaflet, etc. It is better to delegate these tasks to individuals or working groups. The products of these working groups can be discussed later at a full meeting.

The establishing stage can be time for expansion. However, it is also a time when a group can become fixed in its ways and inward-looking. The challenge at this stage is to find ways of keeping the enthusiasm and energy of the members.

Leadership and effective group functioning

How well a group performs depends a great deal on the leadership. Studies of group dynamics point to a wide range of approaches to leadership: these fall along the spectrum shown in Figure 5.7 ranging from a *laissez-faire* ('leave it to the members') approach through to a top-down *authoritarian* ('I am in charge') approach.

authoritarian		democratic		laissez-faire
leader orders group	leader persuades group	leader consults group	leader shares decisions with group	leader leaves decision-making to group

Fig. 5.7 Styles of leadership

The authoritarian approach can reduce creativity and ideas from the members and limit the output of the group. *Laissez-faire* can result in chaos and muddle. The best approach is one where the leader acts as *facilitator* and helps everyone to work together – but when necessary can provide some strong pressure on the group members as a stimulus to action if the meeting has become bogged-down and is failing to reach a decision.

It is helpful to separate out the role of the group leader into two broad areas: *task maintenance functions* are those activities which help to get the group's task done:

setting the agenda
'Today our priority is to plan next year's programme'
introducing new information
'Funds are available for a leaflet'
asking for further information
'How much will this cost?'
making things clear
'I think what Jim means is . . .'
summarizing the present position
'We are now agreed to set up a drama project'
inviting suggestions from members
'Does anyone have any suggestions for how we can . . .?'
prodding
'There's ten minutes left to make a decision on this'
trying to find new ways around a problem
'Let's think again how we can solve this'
reviewing objectives
'Let's remind ourselves that our main aim is to find a way of reaching men with our safe-sex message'
introducing brainstorms, buzz groups (see below)
'Let's try a brainstorm to see if we can get some new ideas'

Group maintenance

Group maintenance functions of a leader are those dealing with the 'well-being' of the group. This might involve:

104

dealing with difficult group members;

encouraging quieter members to participate;

dealing with conflicts;

seeking consensus;

lightening the tension; and

expressing group feelings.

In Chapter 4 the value of participatory learning and group discussion was looked at in some detail. The 'Ten tips for discussion leaders' presented on page 76 suggest how you can encourage group members to take part in discussions. Brainstorming and buzz groups are two more methods that can help improve the effectiveness of groups to make decisions and solve problems.

The *brainstorming* method is an approach for getting a large number of ideas from a group quickly. Suppose you were wishing to think of some possible ideas for a campaign to get the newspapers to publicize accidents in the home. In a typical discussion group, one person suggests an idea and the group discusses it. Then a second person suggests another idea and that is also discussed. At the end of the session you may only have discussed a few suggestions. The quieter persons may have some good ideas but have been too shy to say them aloud. In the brainstorming approach you get the group to generate a list of ideas – and discuss them afterwards.

Brainstorming:

- Place people in a circle and explain to them that you want their ideas and suggestions.
- Emphasize that they should use their imagination and be creative – but no one should comment on each other's suggestions until later.
- Ask one person to write down each suggestion on a large sheet of paper.
- After five or ten minutes you should have a long list of ideas. You can then pick out the ones that look the most useful.

If you want to find solutions to problems more quickly you could always try dividing them into smaller groups and giving a fixed time-limit to produce some suggestions. You may not have enough time for discussion groups and one simple approach is to form *buzz groups*. Ask each member of the group to turn to their neighbour to make small groups of two or three persons. Ask them to discuss the points and give them a time-limit of five minutes to produce some suggestions.

In addition to the suggestions on leadership roles and group discussion methods given above, some guidelines on running successful meetings are listed here.

Things to do to make meetings work

---

1. Prepare an agenda and circulate it with any background papers well in advance.
2. Check out the agenda in advance and make sure you are well prepared.
3. Arrange the seating – make sure it is in a circle.
4. Start the meeting on time.
5. Agree at the beginning on the finishing time – this focuses everybody on the task ahead.
6. Welcome any new members and invite them to introduce themselves.
7. Provide some refreshments if people have come from a long way or the meeting is more than an hour in length.

8. Chair the meeting to ensure order and participation by everyone.
9. Finish on time – if necessary, put off unfinished business to the next meeting.
10. Thank everyone for their contribution.

Patient-education

Patient-education is the name for one-to-one and group education provided to patients in clinics and hospitals as part of the treatment and rehabilitation process. Typical examples of patient-education would be:

- Explaining how much, how often and when medicines should be taken and possible side-effects.
- Special diets, physical exercises that need to be taken for rehabilitation after an illness or operation.
- Advice on diet and self-administering of injections of insulin for diabetic patients.
- Explaining in advance details of an operation in order to reduce patient's anxiety.
- Advice for persons diagnosed to be suffering from an illness, e.g. sickle-cell anaemia, diabetes, etc.
- Explaining to the parents of a dehydrated child how to prepare and give their child oral rehydration solution.

A well-organized patient-education programme can speed up the recovery process, enable a hospital to discharge patients more quickly, release hospital beds and reduce complications and the need for follow-up.

Fig. 5.8 Patient-education

Many examples of health problems can be prevented with effective patient-education. One good example of the need for patient-education is tuberculosis. A person must continue to take medicines for at least six months. Many stop taking medicines once they feel better and the tuberculosis returns.

Another example of a patient-education programme is a nutrition rehabilitation centre where, following diagnosis of malnutrition, the mother is allowed to stay with the child in the hospital. During the child's recovery she is given practical advice on nutrition and child-feeding to prevent the child becoming malnourished again.

Growth monitoring is more than just the regular weighing of children and the detection of slowing of growth. The real importance of growth monitoring is not the weighing itself, but the opportunity provided for education of parents about health, nutrition and child development.

In this chapter, patient-education has been introduced as part of the discussion of face-to-face communication. However, it is also possible to use other approaches. In the South Indian State of Tamil Nadu, a project developed a series of audiocassettes with songs and drama on a range of health topics including nutrition and worms. Other ways for using waiting areas for patient-education include exhibitions, video players, tables with leaflets on different topics and a library of books on self-care and health that can be borrowed by patients (see Figure 5.9).

Steps involved in planning a patient-education programme

---

1. Find out what your intended audience thinks and feels about the health issue. You can apply the concepts introduced in Chapter 2 and identify: important beliefs and the role of culture determining the take-up of the practices; whether there are others in the family or community that should be involved in the patient-education; and whether there are enabling factors such as resources or specific skills that have to be considered.
2. Identify and separate the different learning components of the patient-education, including: what facts need to be explained; the role of decision-making, psychomotor or communication skills; and whether there are any attitudes that should be encouraged, e.g. a positive attitude towards recovery and confidence in one's own ability to cope.
3. Apply the understandings gained in the two steps above and select the most appropriate advice to give (remember the characteristics of good advice given in Figure 3.6).
4. Decide *where* the patient education should take place: in the waiting area, during the consultation, after the consultation, in the hospital ward or at the home of the patient?
5. Decide *who* should do the patient-education – a doctor, nurse, lay counsellor or community health worker?
6. Decide what *method* to use – one-to-one, small group or large meeting; demonstrations, songs, puppet or theatre?
7. Decide what *learning aids* would be required to support the programme – real objects, models; wallcharts, slides, video; 'take-home' reminders such as a leaflet or calendar?
8. Decide how you will *evaluate* the outcome of the patient-education in the short- and long-term.

---

one-to-one
demonstrations
small-group sessions
self-help groups
lay health educators
drama and puppet shows
songs

wall-paintings (murals)
posters
real objects, e.g. foods, improved latrines
audiocassettes/videos in waiting areas
leaflets
lending libraries

**have all been used in health care settings
for patient-education**

Fig. 5.9 Patient-education

Child health clinics can be very noisy places and mothers are often distracted by having to pay attention to their children. One way of dealing with this is to provide a crèche where the children can be looked after for a short period while the mothers attend the patient-education session. Some of the steps in planning a patient-education programme are listed on page 107.

Teaching and learning face-to-face communication skills

Most of the health education and health promotion programmes you undertake will involve some face-to-face communication activities. If you are involving field-staff and volunteers you will probably need to include some training in face-to-face communication. Chapter 4 describes how you can prepare a job description followed up by a task analysis identifying the different kinds of learning involved, including:

- Any *facts* that should be learnt in order to give advice and make decisions.
- How to make any *decisions* required, e.g. planning the patient-education or counselling programme, when to refer the client for a HIV test, for example, how to respond to difficult questions.
- Face-to-face *communication skills* including listening skills, non-verbal communication, asking questions, obtaining feedback, showing empathy, using learning aids.
- *Psycho-motor skills* involved in the face-to-face encounter such as giving an injection, mixing a weaning food.
- *Attitudes*, especially respect, confidentiality, tolerance, patience.

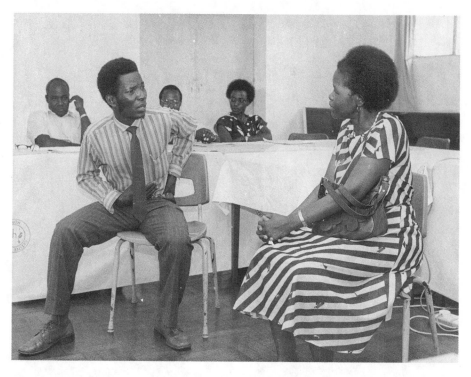

Fig. 5.10 Training health workers in counselling on AIDS in Uganda

One of the best ways of learning communication skills is through role play where the participants act out the one-to-one or group situations and afterwards discuss and learn from their experiences. This can be followed up with practice in real situations in the community under supervision. The use of role-play methods is described in Chapter 4.

Summary

This chapter has looked at ways in which you can improve the effectiveness of your face-to-face communication skills.

1. Both verbal and non-verbal communication have an impact on the effectiveness of face-to-face encounters.
2. Listening is an active process involving asking questions and showing interest and responsiveness.
3. The effectiveness of face-to-face communication depends both on choosing the right time and place for the encounter as well as good communication skills during the actual session.
4. Patient-education should take into account principles of effective face-to-face communication, teaching and learning.
5. Opportunities should be provided for fieldworkers to learn skills in face-to-face communication. The best way to acquire these skills is through role-play followed by practice under supervision in real-life situations.

6. Working with communities

'primary health care starts with people and their health problems, and since they have a major role to play in solving these problems they have to be actively involved in doing just that rather than being passive recipients of care from above.
... it is active involvement that most distinguishes primary health care from the kind of basic health services that were so much looked forward to in the past and that subsequently were so disappointing in practice.
... for people to be intelligently involved in caring for their own health they have to understand what leads to health and what endangers it . . .
... the very first element of primary health care is educating people and communities on health matters.'

Halfdan Mahler, Address to World Health Assembly, 1986

In earlier chapters you saw that many influences on people's behaviour are at the community level. Yet, in the past, health educators have placed too much emphasis on health education with individuals in isolation from their family and community. Many difficulties people face in improving their health, such as poverty, lack of resources and exploitation by others, can only be overcome if people work together for their common good.

The introductory chapter of this book described different approaches to health education. The persuasion approach was contrasted with an informed decision-making approach emphasizing community participation and empowerment. When the idea of primary health care was launched, community participation was one of the most important components. Community participation was also part of the more recent idea of health promotion. But community participation is a term that is not understood very well. Some persons feel that it is given too much emphasis and that it is the 'mythology of the decade'. Although everyone talks about it, community participation is often not put into practice. This chapter will explore different ways of working at the community level for the promotion of health. In particular it will:

1. Explain the concept of community participation, its difference from the conventional 'top-down' planning approaches and the advantages that can come from involving communities in participating in health education programmes.
2. Explore the difficulties encountered in community participation programmes and how these problems can be resolved by careful planning.
3. Examine the role of communication and participatory learning methods in working for change at the community level.

The concept of community participation

The first question that we need to consider is, what does community participation really mean? What do we mean by the community becoming involved and participating in improvement of health?

The word community is used in many different ways. It can be used to describe a *place* or small geographical area; a *group* of people sharing some interest;

111

Fig. 6.1 The top-down approach to planning

or a *social network* of relationships at a local level. So 'community' means more than just people who live close together; it implies sharing and working together in some way. As you will see in a later section, people can live in the same village, but be divided in interests and share little in common.

The term 'community' can also be applied to people who do not live in the same neighbourhood but share characteristics, e.g. youths, prostitutes, an ethnic minority, drug addicts, handicapped persons. An *out-reach approach* is the name that is sometimes used for educational programmes directed at a special group that does not necessarily live in the same neighbourhood.

'Top-down' and 'bottom-up' approaches

One way of defining community participation is to compare it with other approaches which do not involve participation. The traditional approach in health care planning is for the decisions to be made by senior persons in health services – the so-called 'experts'. This approach is sometimes called the 'top-down' approach and contrasted with the 'bottom-up' approach where members of the community make the decisions.

This approach of leaving decisions to professional persons is also used by many health educators. Research may be carried out through surveys to find out what the community thinks and believes to be the problems. But in the end it is usually the health educator who makes the decisions on what goes into the programmes based on medically-defined needs.

Traditional education is often *indoctrination*. Indoctrination is the process of telling people what to do. We make the decisions and expect them to follow. Many people assume that just because they have invited members of the community to a meeting, community participation is taking place. This is not always the case and you will need to look carefully to find out what is really going on. Are the planners using it just to tell the villagers what to do? Or have they come to consult the people and give them a say in their own future?

The term community participation is often applied to programmes where self-help labour is used. The community may contribute labour to dig a latrine

Fig. 6.2 The fact that there is a meeting does not mean that community participation is taking place

for the school in its village. However, is this genuine participation? Are the people doing it because they have been told to do it? Or did they themselves decide to do it?

Spectrum of participation

When we carefully examine different interpretations of the phrase 'community participation' we find that it is used to cover a whole range of very different actions. The American planner Sherry Arnstein suggested that there is a continuum of participation (Figure 6.3). At one extreme there are actions that are really forms of manipulation. Manipulation means controlling people like puppets even though we pretend to let them make decisions.

At the opposite extreme there is total participation or complete control of its affairs by the community. For example we may give the local community control over the health budget for a locality. The community may run the health clinic and make the important decisions. Between these two extremes is a range of other activities that can sometimes happen. One common activity is consultation or asking a community's opinion. However, holding a meeting to ask people's opinions is a very limited form of participation if the final decisions are made by outsiders.

An out-reach programme usually involves sending fieldworkers into communities to work with people who have particular needs, such as young people or drug addicts, etc. The fieldworkers can be health workers or recruited from the target communities themselves. An out-reach approach can be top-down when all the decision-making and priorities are set by the external agency. However it is also possible to use a community participation approach if the target communities and locally-recruited fieldworkers are allowed to participate in decision-making.

113

manipulation	▲	*decision taken by outsiders* *community given impression they* *are involved in decision-making*
consultation	│	*opinion of community sought* *but decision left to outsiders*
community control	▼	*complete power to make decisions given* *to community*

Fig. 6.3 Simplified version of Arnstein's ladder of participation

Projects may say that they are using community participation or involvement and it is important to find out whether this is actually true. David Werner sees community participation as one of the key features that distinguish what he calls 'community supportive' from 'community oppressive' programmes. The list below draws on the work of David Werner, Susan Rifkin and Patricia Martin and presents a checklist of questions you can apply to find out how much participation is really taking place.

A checklist of questions for finding the degree of participation in a programme

---

- Is the community involved in planning, management and control of the health programme at the community level?
- Were the felt needs of the community found out at the outset of the programme and was notice taken of them in planning the programme objectives?
- What forms of social organization exist in the community and to what extent have they been involved in the decision-making process (e.g. farmer's cooperatives, clubs, churches, political organizations, trade unions, etc.)?
- Is there a mechanism for dialogue between health system personnel and community leadership?
- Is there a mechanism for community representatives to be involved in decision-making at higher levels and is this effective?
- Is there any evidence of the external agents changing their plans as a result of criticism from the community?
- Are deprived groups, such as poor, landless, unemployed, and women, adequately represented in the decision-making process?
- Are local resources used, such as labour, buildings, money?
- Was the community involved in evaluating the project and in the drafting of the final report?

What benefits come from community participation?

Many people find it unnecessary to justify community participation. They see it as a fundamental right and part of the process of democracy. However, as you will see later in the chapter, genuine community participation must be planned in advance and will require extra time and effort. You may need to persuade others of the benefits from community participation to get funding and support.

Justifications for community participation come from a variety of sources, including lessons learned from the failures of conventional 'top-down' educational programmes as well as the achievements of community-based programmes.

The need for a community approach

An important justification for community participation is the need to shift the emphasis from the individual to the community. In earlier chapters you will have seen that many influences on a behaviour are at the community level and not under the control of individuals. These include social pressure from other people through norms, shared culture and the local socio-economic situation. Even when the influences are at the national level, it is often through pressure from communities that governments will change.

Here are listed some of the different kinds of groups that you might already find in the community or may start up yourself as a result of your community participation programme.

Types of community groups

Self-help groups
Run by people for their own benefit, e.g. cooperatives, baby clubs.
Representative groups
Elected and answerable to the community – such as community associations.
Pressure groups
A group of self-appointed citizens taking action on what they see to be the interests of the whole community – such as putting on pressure to improve the school, get garbage collected, do something about a dangerous road.
Traditional organizations
Well-established groups, usually meeting the needs of a particular section of the community – Rotary Club, mother's union, parent-teachers' association, church group.
Social groups
Exist mainly to put on social events – e.g. sports clubs, music groups, carnival group.
Welfare groups
Exist to improve welfare for others – e.g. run feeding programmes.

Drawing on local knowledge

Communities often have detailed knowledge about their surroundings. This 'community environmental knowledge' includes plants, animals, water sources, building materials, and treatment and prevention of disease. It makes sense to involve communities in making plans because they know local conditions and the possibilities for change.

Making programmes locally relevant and acceptable

A major problem in the development of health services is the gap between the decision-makers and the community. A common complaint is that their projects are not supported and maintained by the community. However, usually the community was never consulted. If the community is involved in choosing priorities and deciding on plans it is much more likely to become involved in the programme and take up the services because they are seen to be meeting their needs. The timings and location will be more appropriate to the community who will then be more likely to use them.

115

A good example of the importance of community participation comes from the experiences of water-supply programmes where the community can participate in choosing the best location of water taps, providing labour in the initial construction, ensuring that the water systems are used properly and in the setting-up of a community organization for reporting break-downs and carrying out simple maintenance. The cartoons in this chapter are all taken from The World Health Organization's excellent manual *Achieving Success in Water and Sanitation*.

Developing self-reliance, self-confidence, empowerment and problem-solving skills

The enthusiasm that comes from community participation can lead to a greater sense of self-reliance for the future. For example, communities are usually willing to participate in water programmes because they see that benefits will come. The feeling of community solidarity and self-reliance from participating in decisions over their own future through a water project can lead to further activities.

Better relationship between health worker and community

Community participation leads to a better relationship between the community and health workers. Instead of a servant–master relationship, there is trust and partnership.

Primary health care

The Alma Ata Declaration on Primary Health Care in 1978 extended the notion of appropriate health care beyond that of simply providing decentralized services. It also considered the need to tackle economic and social causes of ill-health. In the quote at the beginning of this chapter, Halfdane Mahler drew from his experiences as Director of WHO to explain how health education and community participation are essential (and often missing!) ingredients of primary health care.

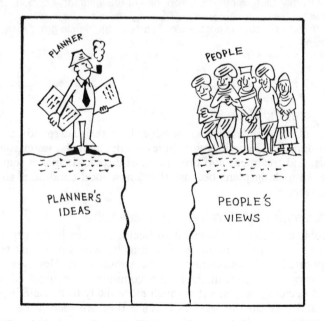

Fig. 6.4 Bridging the gap between planners and the community

116

Emphasizes community rather than individuals.
Makes programmes relevant to local situation.
Ensures community motivation and support.
Improves take-up of services.
Promotes self-help and self-reliance.
Improves communication between health workers and community.
Enables the development of primary health care.

Concept of needs

Before proceeding further, we need to examine critically the concept of needs and the implications this has for the process of community participation. Basing a health programme on a community's felt needs is often criticized by planners and health workers. They often object and claim that the members of the community are not really able to define their own needs. However, this raises fundamental questions. What do we mean by needs? In reality, there is no such thing as the 'real need' for a particular community but a range of perspectives.

- *Felt needs* are what people 'feel' or their 'wants'. They may only be the feelings of individual people or a collective feeling shared by the whole group.
- *Expressed needs* have not only been felt but have been expressed – brought to the attention of the authorities by requests, petitions or complaints, etc.
- *Agency-determined needs* are what external services, such as health workers and planners, have decided the community needs; they do not necessarily correspond to felt needs.

Many 'community participation' programmes are really 'top-down' and based on agency-determined needs. However, imposing our views on communities is dangerous because we do not always understand the whole situation. It also represents a rejection of the community's right to determine its own needs. Also, if the community has other needs which it feels are more important, it is unlikely to take action on the agency-determined needs.

Felt needs are based on people's judgements of their present situation and possibilities for change. These judgements may depend on beliefs about the extent and nature of health problems, and their causes and possibilities for prevention and cure. These beliefs are influenced by their previous experience, education, understanding of epidemiology and biology. So felt needs may be based on a realistic assessment of their situation by the community. But they can also be based on misunderstandings and incomplete knowledge.

For example, many communities think of health as a product of doctors and medicines. They are more likely to define their felt needs in terms of wanting health facilities and curative services rather than preventive measures.

- *Felt needs* include a person's or community's assessment of the present situation and potential for change;
- *which may depend on beliefs* about the extent and nature of health problems, their causes and possibilities for prevention and cure; and
- *are influenced by previous experience*, culture, education, understanding of epidemiology and biology.

117

Another problem in community participation comes with the concept of community itself. We often assume that everyone in a village or community agrees with each other and shares the same felt needs. This is not always the case. Societies may be divided according to inequalities in wealth, power and employment. These inequalities are often called 'social stratification' (literally the 'layering' of the community). Other forms of divisions can exist according to religion, language, tribe or race.

People may disagree with each other. It can be very difficult to get everyone to agree at public meetings over what they want. Frequently the needs that emerge from meetings are those of the dominant powerful groups. The needs of disadvantaged sections of the community such as the poor or women may be ignored. For example, a recent review of community participation in family

Fig. 6.5 You can easily be misled if you do not understand the divisions in a community

THE FIELD WORKER	THE COMMUNITY RESPONSE
Ask the community about its problems and needs	
	community explains its needs
Ask questions to find out basis of needs	
	community explains basis of its needs
Respect community needs but also challenge it to consider wider issues and provide educational inputs	
	community acquires awareness of other issues and begins to consider alternative needs

Fig. 6.6 The process of dialogue in community participation

118

planning projects in Asia describes how the various local committees consisted mainly of male elders. A criticism of the nationwide community development programme set up in India in the 1950s is that village *panchayat* committees were dominated by high-caste, landowning, and better-off men.

So community participation is not simply a passive process of responding to needs of the community but an *active process* of working with groups to define needs. This should be based on dialogue, sharing of understanding and ensuring that the needs that are acted upon are based on informed decision-making and represent the interests of all sections of the community. This process of dialogue is shown in Figure 6.6 which is loosely based on the work of Batten.

Community participation as a process

Community participation cannot be achieved through occasional visits and holding meetings. You should allow a realistic time scale for your programme. It should be seen as a **process** over time that can go through a series of overlapping stages such as those shown in Figure 6.7.

entry: getting to know the community	*Learning about the community, its structure and pattern; initial contacts with families, leaders and community groups; discussions on concerns and felt needs.*
initial actions	*Action on achievable, short-term aims based on felt needs which bring the community together and build confidence.*
further activities and organization-building	*Strengthening of community organization; formation of committees; educational inputs; selection of community members for training as lay workers; decision-making on priorities; further actions.*
evaluation and reflection	*Reflection on achievements. Decisions about future activities. Reduction in dependence on external project and greater community involvement in future activities.*

Fig. 6.7 Stages in community participation programmes

Entry: getting to know the community

The starting point for any community-based activity is to get to know the community. You will need to identify and have informal discussion with opinion leaders, community groups, fieldworkers from government and non-governmental organizations. It is helpful to make a *profile* of the community in order to identify any special features which will affect the success of community participation programmes. It is important to know of any previous health programmes that may have taken place in that area – and whether they were successes or failures.

You should try to find out what the community feels are its needs. It may already have brought some of them to the attention of health and other services

Fig. 6.8 It's important to look for existing institutions that might be built upon in community participation programmes

through complaints and letters. If not, you will have to meet individuals and groups to find out their felt needs. It is important to know whether the whole community agrees on its needs or if there are differences. Are there minorities with different needs? Are there conflicting interests?

Listed here is a range of different kinds of information that you might find useful in planning your programme. The data required will depend on the health issues you are interested in, the special features of the locality. You should also consult with the community over the kinds of information to collect.

Information required for making the community profile

Environment: geography, urban/rural, transport, land use, recreational facilities, housing.

History: history of area, activities of local groups, issues that the community have expressed concern about in the past; previous government and NGO activities on health; previous history of community action.

General data: total population, age distribution, children under 14 years, population 65 years, under-fives, turnover of population, birth rate, family sizes, vulnerable groups, e.g. single-parent families and handicapped, ethnic groups, religion, social class, employment.

Health and other services: utilization of hospitals/clinics/private doctors, traditional healers; social services, agriculture, community development, adult education, schools; other government services; relationships with community and other agencies; degree of conflict and cooperation between agencies.

Perceptions of area: residents' perceptions of problems of area; attitudes towards other residents, agencies, officials, local politicians, attitudes and beliefs concerning health and felt needs for health education and health care services.

Community structure, norms and traditions: networks of information, influence and care; family structure; opinion leaders, divisions and conflicts; power structure;

120

norms that determine people's attitudes to taking action to achieve some change; norms that govern the role of women; norms that govern health and illness behaviour.

Organizations: religious organizations; women's groups, youth groups, non-governmental organizations;

Communications: local newspapers, newsletter, notice boards, radio, television.

Power and leadership: existing community organizations, committees, etc., businesses; trade unions; elected politicians; political parties; local political forums, such as ward councils; officials in health services, housing and education, etc.

In any community there will always be individuals with special influence. These opinion leaders may be chiefs, religious leaders, teachers or older persons. It is important to find out who are the opinion leaders and what *they* think are the needs of the community. They can help you in many ways – but beware of being misled (see Figure 6.5)!

The contribution of local leaders to community health education

---

1. Bring people to meetings.
2. Arrange for and find meeting places.
3. Help reach more people by telling others.
4. Help people in the community know you and gain confidence in you.
5. Give general information about the programme and help interpret it to the people.
6. Help identify problems and resources in the community.
7. Help plan and organize programmes and community activities.
8. Help plan and organize any services that might be provided.
9. Give simple demonstrations.
10. Conduct meetings.
11. Lead youth groups and various individual projects.
12. Interest others in becoming leaders.
13. Help neighbours learn skills.
14. Share information with neighbours.
15. Serve as an officer in an organization or chairperson of a committee.

(Adapted from Peace Corps (1978), *Community Health Education in Developing Countries – Getting Started*)

Initial actions

Building up community participation may involve meeting individuals to find out about the problems of the area. It also involves working with large groups. It is usual to have community meetings early in the programme. These provide an opportunity for everybody to participate in the discussion. But you should carefully prepare yourself to deal with questions and problems that might arise, and if people are going to bring up an issue such as roads or the state of the local school that is outside your own control, you can then invite persons from those departments to join in the discussion.

How you proceed will depend a great deal on the power structure of the community and the presence of divisions and opposing interests. Some of the

	Community structure	Your response
(1)	One main group with single leader	*Work with the single organization and leader*
(2)	Two groups (in this case one larger than the other)	*Find point of agreement between the two groups*
(3)	Community divided into more than two factions	*Find point of agreement between the groups.*
(4)	No distinct structures or divisions (e.g. newly-occupied area which has not yet developed a social structure)	*Identify issues that will encourage people to come together and encourage formation of community structures and emergence of leadership.*

Fig. 6.9 Community power structures

ways communities can be split into factions are shown in Figure 6.9. How do you think your approach might differ with each of the community structures?

With only one faction in the community as in (1) you will need to work with that single group and its leader. With situations (2) and (3) where there are two or more factions it is more difficult and you will have to balance the needs of different groups and avoid appearing to favour one group over another. You will have to find areas of common interest that the groups can agree on.

Most rural communities will have well-developed social structures. However the situation in urban areas can be quite different and resemble (4). If there are no distinct groups, such as in a newly-created housing settlement, your priority should be to encourage some kind of community structure to develop. You can do this by finding an issue that everyone is concerned about enough to attend meetings and take action.

These early decisions on issues and actions will have an important influence on future developments. A successful outcome will build up confidence. You should encourage the community to select short-term achievable objectives that will unite different factions in common action.

Further activities and organization-building

The success of this initial action should result in the community seeing the benefits of working together, gaining more confidence and attracting more people to join in activities. The need for some structure will become apparent. Out of the large meeting, a small group is often formed, such as a village water committee. You can work closely with these small groups and advise them on the best way to organize themselves and help to resolve any internal tensions and conflicts.

As the community begins to develop trust and confidence in you, it will be prepared to listen to your suggestions for further actions. Individuals in the community will begin to acquire new skills as a result of their involvement and will identify needs for further education. You should continue your dialogue and provide educational inputs in response to their interests. As their perspectives broaden, they will be prepared to tackle wider issues. You should take a less active role and encourage the community to take more responsibility for maintaining the project.

Evaluation and reflection

As activities progress, you should keep a record of achievements so that you can evaluate the programme. The local community can share in evaluation of the programme through collecting data and providing support for survey teams. Results of any evaluation can be discussed with the community who should be given an opportunity to reflect on their achievements and share in the making of longer-term plans for their area.

The big test for any community participation programme is whether activities continue once external support is reduced. Activities will continue or collapse depending on the strength of the community structures created during the early activities.

These stages should not be applied in a rigid way. They should be seen as overlapping components of a process of working with communities. Whether or not you have to go through them depends on the situation in the community and what has already happened. In some situations there will already be a range of community-based activities that you can build upon. In other communities there may be few activities and divisions or conflicts and you need to start by building up community organization.

Participatory learning and education for critical awareness

It is important to build learning experiences into community participation pro-grammes. In this way, the community will be able to understand more about the different factors that influence their health and how these factors can be changed. But the approach to teaching should be quite different from traditional health education where the teacher is the 'expert' and the community is expected to accept what it is told and often made to feel inferior. It is important to use methods that develop a critical awareness of the situation and *empower* the community to work together for change.

The Brazilian adult educator/priest Paulo Freire has been an influential critic of traditional formal educational approaches. He was deeply critical of traditional approaches to education which he compared with depositing facts in people's heads, rather like money in a bank. Instead, he calls for a problem-posing approach involving dialogue on an equal basis between the community and the educator.

In problem-posing education people develop their power to perceive critically the way they exist in the world with which and in which they find themselves; they come to see the world not as a static reality but as a reality in process, in transformation.

Paulo Freire

The special name he uses for this approach to education is '*conscientization*' or consciousness-raising. In this approach, the community is encouraged to *critically reflect* on their situation and how they might transform it through action. The process of learning from action he called 'praxis'.

123

Participatory learning methods have already been discussed in Chapter 4 and characteristics of educational methods for promoting empowerment are shown here, adapted from the work of Susan Kindervatter.

Characteristics of learning methods for empowerment

- Opportunities built in for discussion, feedback and participation.
- Methods used usually involve simulations, role-plays and problem-solving exercises: learning aids such as flannelgraphs and pictures are used that can promote discussion.
- Less emphasis is put on acquisition of specific knowledge and more on development of problem-solving skills, critical thinking, reflection and analysis.
- Uses small groups (less than 20).
- Open-ended with objectives determined by the whole group.
- Trainer acts as facilitator to process rather than teacher and 'expert'.

Paulo Freire's method was to prepare pictures of every-day situations and difficulties. These were shown to the community which was then asked to discuss and critically reflect on them. Others, such as the Laedza Batanani Theatre Group in Botswana, have followed his approach, using drama instead of pictures. In their programme, a theatre group visited communities and developed the drama from local issues. Following presentation of the drama, the community was involved in discussion of the issues and suggesting solutions. It was possible to stop the drama at different stages and ask for comments and suggestions or for the community to take part. Another approach is to use members of the community as actors and let them base the content of the drama on their experiences. Chapter 7 will give more examples of theatre for community participation.

Many people are only used to traditional formal one-way teaching. They can find it threatening to have discussion and criticism in the session. So it is important to provide training in participatory learning methods to fieldworkers in community-based projects.

Using lay workers and volunteers

Any information about health that you give the community will be passed on to others through informal contacts. We can deliberately encourage this process by selecting members of the community and giving them training as 'peer health educators'. An approach that is now used in many primary health programmes is to encourage communities to select one of their number to receive simple training as village health workers or community health workers. They can become highly effective communicators because they share the same background characteristics as their fellow-villagers.

Two approaches have been used for selection of lay persons for training. In 'out-reach' projects, the health education agency appoints the lay persons. They may have been selected as a result of having been identified as 'opinion leaders' or through a process such as advertising and recruiting from a public meeting. However, in programmes that emphasize community participation, it is best to ask the community to select one or more of their members for training as a lay health educator. With the expansion in interest in primary health care there have

124

Fig. 6.10 Village health worker

been many experiments using community health workers, and evaluations have suggested the guidelines shown here.

Guidelines for using lay workers in community health programmes

---

- The persons selected should match the project's needs. If you are trying to reach youths, then train young people as 'peer educators'. If you are working with women, use women of an age similar to that of the target groups.
- Select people who are already respected in the community. They may be people who are leading figures in the community programmes, traditional birth attendants, traditional healers or other respected persons.
- Involve the community in the selection of the volunteers. Brief them on the kinds of personal qualities that are needed of trustworthiness, acceptability, skill in communication and educational background.
- Provide a training that is practical and includes participatory learning methods.
- Provide regular support and follow-up to encourage the volunteers in their work. Give them opportunities to share their problems with you and the other volunteers.

Planning for community participation

You have seen that community participation can bring considerable benefits to health programmes. However, overcoming the problems described above and achieving community participation require careful planning.

125

Involvement of other sectors

The community may bring up needs that cannot be met by the health services. For example, Tumwine described in 1989 how he and his colleagues recognized a high incidence of schistosomiasis in a rural Zimbabwe village and were planning to motivate the community to build and use improved latrines. He asked the people what their main problems were. He expected the response 'Schistosomiasis', but to his surprise, they answered 'food' and a disease whose description fitted pellagra. The team ended up discussing drought, relief food and food production.

If your own programme is not very flexible and cannot follow this example, it would be important to involve persons from other departments such as agriculture, rural development and adult literacy. If they are involved, they can act on social and economic needs and you can concentrate on meeting the felt needs that are specific to health. But health, social and economic needs are all inter-related, so it is important that you work as a team.

If your activities only involve a single health topic, such as AIDS, water, nutrition, sanitation or immunization you may find that these are not the most important issues to the community. In that case you should try to involve other health workers in the initial activities.

Initial briefings

It is important that everyone involved in implementing the programme meets and carefully considers all the implications of a community participation strategy. Outside professionals such as engineers and planners may see themselves as the experts and not recognize that the community should have a say in their affairs. The health workers in the community may feel threatened by allowing people in the community to make decisions. Everyone involved should be made aware of the advantages of letting communities decide for themselves what their priorities should be.

Time-scale for community participation

Another serious problem comes from the short time-scale of many projects. It is not enough to make a single visit to a community and expect that everyone will join and work together. You have seen that community participation is a *process* that takes time to develop. Unfortunately many health programmes are planned on a short time-scale. A 'project cycle' of two or three years is common. At the end of this period sponsors are often demanding 'results' such as completed latrines or decreases in morbidity. However, it is extremely difficult to develop genuine community participation in such a short time. Although lip-service may be paid to community participation, projects often dispense with that in the rush to meet targets.

Open-ended community-oriented objectives

When setting objectives for your programmes, it is important not to be too rigid on your desired outcomes. If you are genuinely promoting community participation your objectives will be determined by the community themselves. This must be pointed out to any donor agencies who should not try to impose objectives on the community. Keep your objectives open-ended.

As the main point of community participation is to develop self-reliance, critical awareness and problem-solving skills in communities, this should be

Fig. 6.11 Community participation is often dispensed with in the rush to get the job done

reflected in the objectives. Look at the two sets of objectives below. What differences can you see in them?

1. By the end of the programme 20 pit latrines will have been dug.
2. By the end of the programme the community would have come together to consider how they might work together to improve their community and have started on a topic of their own choice.

The first objective is based on changes in a specific health behaviour. The second objective is concerned with changes *in people* rather than particular behaviours. These 'process' objectives deal with more fundamental changes such as self-awareness, self-empowerment and problem-solving skills.

Evaluation of community participation programmes

Evaluation involves showing that the objectives have been achieved in the most efficient manner possible. Evaluation of community participation programmes should be based, not only on achievement of specific health and behaviour changes, but also on achievement of the 'process objectives' described above.

If you take community participation seriously, the community should be involved in the evaluation of the programme as well. Evaluation becomes a learning experience in which everybody looks at what has been achieved and decides what more needs to be done. There is growing interest in *participatory evaluation* and *action-research* that are described further in the final chapter of this book.

In practice, evaluation has to fulfil several distinct needs. You may be mainly concerned with looking at achievements, the effectiveness of your methods and whether the community has found it worthwhile. However, your employers may not understand – or be sympathetic to – the full implications of community participation and may not accept the value of outcomes that the community feels are important.

127

It is a good idea to include a range of indicators in the evaluation schedule that take into account both the community's as well as other key groups' interests. You can compare changes in your target community with 'control' communities where the programme is not operating. A good programme will respond to the community's needs with a flexible evaluation which adjusts to changing situations.

Need for community-based field organizers

Your community may already be united with a clear idea of its needs and an organized structure with which you can work. Then your task is an easy one. However, the initial situation is often a community divided in its interests and felt needs and poorly organized to take advantage of available resources. In that case, establishing dialogue, bringing people together, discussing felt needs and resolving conflicts will require time, effort and skill. You will need to decide who will carry out these demanding tasks. If you cannot do this yourself, you will have to involve others.

One approach is to obtain the funds to employ a special group of workers. However, while it is helpful to have full-time community workers, community participation should not be seen as something that can only be done when a programme has full-time community workers on its staff. It should be possible to train health and other fieldworkers and adjust work schedules so that community organization activities are built into their normal workload. Yet most health workers based in clinics and health centres receive little training on methods for working with communities.

Whoever you use to be your community organizers, they must be properly selected and trained to enable them to carry out their task effectively. Their training should enable them to understand community structures; identify opinion leaders; be good listeners and communicators; work with individuals and groups; advise on community organization; and use participatory learning methods.

Summary – conditions for successful community participation programmes

The most important resources for the promotion of health are the people themselves. Through community participation you can use that resource to improve the health of the people. However, it would be wrong to claim that community participation can overcome all the problems facing communities. Some health educators have been criticized for emphasizing community participation while ignoring action to deal with international forces, government policies, natural disasters, poverty and exploitation. These can only be tackled at national and international level. Effective health education cannot ignore politics.

Community participation is not always a feasible strategy. You may not have the time or have access to other fieldworkers for the demanding task of working with local communities, holding dialogue or supporting community organizations, etc. Then you may have no choice but to use approaches such as radio. In urban areas, your target group may be scattered throughout the city so it is not feasible to bring them together for common action and an out-reach approach may be best. In emergencies, such as an epidemic, there simply may not be the time for going through the process of community participation.

However, in most situations a genuine community participation approach is both desirable and feasible – *but can only be achieved if you plan for it*. This involves considering the problems and solutions that have been discussed in this chapter and are summarized opposite.

- Brief all staff on community participation.
- Involve all the relevant agencies.
- Base the programme on an understanding of the local community and their felt needs.
- Have open-ended objectives.
- Have a realistic time-scale.
- Allow genuine community control.
- Use well-trained field-workers.
- Provide support and training for volunteer lay workers.
- Build in dialogue and participatory learning experiences.
- Involve the community in evaluation.

7. Communication – the people's way!

Long before the coming of mass media, great religions and social ideas spread to millions of people by word of mouth. Many communities, even today, learn from, trust and enjoy the spoken word and visual image. In this chapter I will:

1. Look at a range of 'folk' or 'popular' media and consider their potential for communicating health.
2. Consider what needs to be attended to in mobilizing popular media for health education and health promotion.

What are popular media?

Traditional media that appear on special occasions and are only watched by a minority are an important part of a nation's history. But they are not really popular media in the sense that I will deal with in this chapter. The most important characteristic of popular media is that they are enjoyed *today*. They are *living* traditions, enjoyed by many people. Their popularity stems from the following.

- Their entertainment value.
- Their coverage of ideas and issues of universal concern such as love, marriage, honour, failure, success, jealousy, revenge, wealth, poverty, power, family and group conflicts and religion.
- The fact that even though they are based on tradition, they change and adapt to deal with new situations and incorporate the issues and concerns of the day.

Before dealing with different forms of folk media in more detail, let us consider some examples of different popular media.

- The **Calypso** is a type of song that has become highly popular in the Caribbean both through live performances, radio broadcasts and on records. The music has a fast popular beat and contains words that comment on current issues. They often criticize government actions and make fun of national institutions.
- The **Ramlilas** in India take place every year in many villages. Members of the community participate in acting out scenes from the Ramayana, the Hindu epic poem that describes the life of Rama and his battle with evil in the form of the demon-king Ravana. The performances, often in the open air, involve the whole community.
- **Ngonjera** is a form of written and spoken poetry in the local Kiswahili language that became popular in Tanzania in the early 1970s. Two or three actors act out the poem which is often on political or social events. Media such as charts, photographs and real objects are often incorporated. Poetry is so popular that many Swahili newspapers reserve a page for readers' poems.
- In the 1960s among the Tiv people in Nigeria a new style of theatre, **Kwagh-hir**, evolved, combining traditional and ritual elements with a storyteller, acrobats, dancers, puppet-shows, stories and tales. In open-air performances, themes dealing with traditionalism and modernization are performed. The Tiv

people also use singing, dancing, music, drama and story-telling in their rituals, feasts and leisure activities to express their traditions. For many years the drumbeats of 'talking drums' were used to communicate over hundreds of miles and many people today still understand this language. In their music, the rhythms of the drumbeats can communicate messages to the audience.

- In the state of Kerala in Southern India trucks are elaborately decorated with *folk paintings* and *proverbs*. The decorations vary from elaborate and intricate flower designs to characters from Western cartoons.
- The *merolicos* in Mexico are medicine-men who set up stalls at markets and other public places and use ventriloquism, mind-reading, snake-handling and other arts to sell medicinal products. They are treated with respect by the community. The medicine men communicate information about health in their performance.
- In West African towns and villages important announcements are traditionally made by a *town-crier*.

Folk media that have been used in health education include:

- *storytelling*   oral or written
- *drama*   theatre as performance
                  participatory theatre
                  puppets
- *song*   'pop' songs
                  folk songs
- *pictures*   'art'
                  cloth designs

Storytelling

Storytelling is a good way to communicate health.

- stories build on the impact of the spoken word – which is always more powerful than the written word;
- everyone is interested in stories; they can identify themselves with the characters;
- while educated people have been trained to think in a logical, organized way, the story-format is closer to the way most people think;
- people remember information better when it is presented in a story-format than a formal talk or lecture;
- stories can make truth concrete – abstract ideas can be expressed in everyday terms;
- stories begin from things that people understand;
- stories can allow people to discover principles for themselves.

The health topic might form the main story. Another approach is to have the main story dealing with topics that have a high universal appeal, that might be intrigues, quarrels, sexual liaisons, arguments, encounters with ghosts or magic and include health issues as a sub-theme.

A well-developed story will provoke a response if people see it to be relevant to their lives. It should be told in an interesting way, changing one's voice to suit the different characters. The audience should be involved along the way with questions such as, 'Now what do you think happened next?' If people believe in the story and identify themselves with the characters they are more likely to remember the message and take action to change their situation and adopt health-promoting behaviours.

David Hilton describes how the Ladin Gabas Rural Health Programme in Nigeria used the following approach to train village health workers with stories:

1. The teacher tells the story to the class from memory then asks the class questions afterwards to see what they have learned.
2. One student is chosen to repeat the story aloud and the teacher and other students comment.
3. The class then divides into groups of four or five, each of whom then tells the story to his or her group until all have had a chance.
4. Each group then creates a drama from the stories with the students each acting a part.
5. The class comes together and each group presents its drama, which is then discussed, to the class.
6. The class evaluates the performance of each group and if desired chooses the best.

Drama and popular theatre

Drama (sometimes called 'popular theatre') can also be used to promote community participation. It is a powerful way of carrying out Paulo Freire's approach to education that was described in the previous chapter.

In one approach, a drama group visits a community and develops the drama from local issues. Following presentation of the drama the community is involved in discussing issues and suggesting solutions. It is possible to stop the drama at different stages and ask for comments, suggestions or for the community to take part. You do not need professional actors and can develop a performance entirely using local community members where the process of development of the drama becomes as important as the actual performance.

A well-known example of the use of drama in this participatory way is the Laedza Batanani theatre project that was carried out between 1974 and 1977 in Botswana. The name means in the local language, 'The sun is already up – it is time to come and work together.' Its purpose was to present issues through an entertainment medium and 'wake people up' to take collective action to deal with them. They identify three stages in their approach to using drama: problem-identification, drama-scripting and performance.

In the *problem-identification* stage the fieldworkers held workshops where a committee of elders in the community was selected and between 60 and 100 community members were invited. Small-group 'brainstorming' sessions were held (see Chapter 5). These produced a list of ideas from the community which could be grouped into five major categories: village development problems; family problems; value conflicts and social problems; economic concerns; and consumer concerns. The members of the community were asked to put the problems in order of importance and improvise short drama sketches to illustrate them.

The next stage, *drama-scripting*, involved working with the persons selected by the village committee to be the actors. The actors developed the script from the ideas that had been generated earlier. They added a set of characters, such as a miner, a drunkard, or grandmother, to produce a script that was entertaining but still contained key development messages.

The final stage of *performance* took place in villages and at festivals. Following each performance the actors asked the audiences to join them in small-group

132

Fig. 7.1 Theatre group in Zambia

Fig. 7.2 Theatre for development in Botswana

discussion and posed the questions:

Are the problems shown in the drama real problems in your village?
How can these problems be solved?
Does the theatre project help you to overcome the problems?

Their performances also included music and dancing. Simple books were produced based on the stories in the drama and these were given out to audiences and schools. Videotapes were made of performances and these were also found to stimulate discussion.

The Liwonde Primary Health Care Unit in Malawi provides a good example of how drama can be used as part of a primary health care programme. In 1985 their theatre team visited the Mwima community to find out their grievances. These included: absence of a nurse/clinical officer; lack of good protected water; lack of a proper market; various diseases such as diarrhoea, measles and scabies; and hospitals too far away.

After analyzing their research-findings, the team prepared a drama sketch about the location of wells in the village. The play was performed in the village *bwalo*, a square in front of the headman's house that is the traditional place for meetings. The actors did not use real objects but used mime and gestures to create in the audience's imagination features such as houses, goats, a well, a rubbish dump and babies' nappies.

The performance involved the community by directly addressing the audience on controversial issues. For example, when the actor playing a villager complained to the other actor playing the headman about animals fouling the well, the question was put to the audience, 'Is that true? Is that how the well is supposed to be kept?' The audience responded actively, arguing with the actors and each other about the factual and moral issues raised in the play. Since issues about water and wells in rural Malawian society are traditionally the responsibility of women, women were involved in the discussions. Following the drama and a repeat performance, the villagers agreed to work together to improve the well.

This success stimulated the villagers' enthusiasm for primary health care and the health project followed this up with a play about the election of village health committees and the importance of community participation in matters of health. Ten villages in the area formed village health committees which, supported by further drama sketches, actively promoted preventive measures. Topics covered included cementing of wells, chlorinating of wells, promotion of pit latrines and provision of basic medicines such as chloroquine, aspirin and antibiotic eye-ointment.

The success of the theatre programme in these villages led to the use of theatre in other communities. The Primary Health Care Unit held a five-day workshop to train other village health committee members in other communities on the use of theatre for primary health care. This led to an expansion of theatre activities. An evaluation of the theatre programme was carried out in the two areas where extensive use had been made of theatre methods. Between 1985 and 1987, there had been an increase in latrines built and a reduction in diarrhoea. But there had been little change during that same period in a similar area where there had been no drama activities.

Mime is a form of theatre acted out without words. This is of special value when there are many languages in a community. Since 1968 the Jagran theatre company in India has worked in Delhi's slum colonies, performing to audiences of up to 2000 people. With 14 languages and many hundred dialects, spoken theatre is almost impossible in these colonies but the language of mime communicates to all on the street or a village immediately.

Jagran have described their approach as follows:

The Jagran troupe performs in the midst of slums and villages in various states of India. It is an informal affair. The message goes round by word of mouth.

And it is a matter of minutes for crowds to assemble around the troupe. On the surface the show is entertainment, humorous and light-hearted. The audience laugh at themselves. They laugh at the drunkard, at the villain who insists on dowry, at the fellow who eats dirty food and suffers from diarrhoea. But beneath the slapstick and comedy are messages aimed to make the audience view their lives in a different perspective. The actors are members of the audience, dressed like them; but for the grease paint, the comic situations are theirs and so are the tragedies. And with all this identification, communication becomes almost complete.

One of Jagran's plays is called *The Monster of Malnutrition*. The father and son are scared by a huge monster. They discover that this is due to their eating habits, so they change their diet to a healthy, balanced one and are able to kill off the monster. The facts of nutrition are introduced in a comical, humorous way so the audience are entertained but do not forget the point.

Puppets

Puppets are a form of drama with considerable potential for health education. Puppets may be part of the tradition of a country such as the Punch and Judy shown in Britain and the shadow puppets of Indonesia. One advantage of puppets is that it is possible for them to say things on sensitive topics that it would be unacceptable for an actor to say in a drama. People will accept puppets criticizing traditions and institutions. So puppets are particularly valuable for dealing with controversial topics such as sex education and AIDS. In the USA they have been used to reduce the fear and anxiety that children have about going to stay in hospital or visiting the dentist.

- Different types of puppets are: *glove puppets* with heads made from papier mâché or clay; *rod puppets* with figures on wooden rods; *paper-bag puppets* with faces drawn on paper bags; *jointed puppets* moved by string; and *shadow puppets* where a cardboard cutout casts a large shadow against a wall.
- Don't just wave the puppets around: make them do things – chase, nod, fight, hit and even kiss! Practise the movements in front of a mirror – or ask people to watch and give advice on your performance.
- Give the puppets names, special clothing and personalities. Lighten the tension by including humour. Include music and songs. Keep it simple – do not try to cover too much. Entertain – avoid preaching.
- You can make a proper stage that can be easily put up and taken down again for transportation. However, a wall or curtain for the puppeteers to stand behind is usually enough. A large piece of cloth can be hung across two trees or across a doorway or the window of a house.
- Choose the timing of the performances carefully. Find out when your audience – women, children or men – are free. Choose suitable locations. Markets, festivals, agricultural shows, health committee meetings or schools all provide good opportunities to use puppets. Make sure performances are well-publicized in advance.

Many people see puppets as being relevant only for children and are surprised when they realize how useful they can be with adults. For example, in the Laedza Batanani theatre project in Botswana, a puppet show was given to entertain the children on the mornings of the theatre performances and the adults were also interested. They found that controversial village persons, such as the traditional healer, could be portrayed without giving offence, by using puppets.

Fig. 7.3 Puppets

As with drama, puppets have most impact when the community participates in the preparation of the programme, performing the show and can discuss it afterwards. Even so, puppets can be filmed and broadcast on television and provide entertaining and interesting health education to large audiences. The American programme *Sesame Street* uses a format of real actors, puppets and songs to provide a valuable educational experience and has been watched by millions of pre-school children throughout the world.

For further ideas on using puppets you can consult the excellent handbook *Puppets for Health* by Gill and Sue Gordon based on their extensive field experience in the Bawkur District of Ghana (see Appendix A).

Songs

The words and music of songs can have a powerful effect on the emotions. Musicians carry great influence and are admired and looked up to. Songs can be used to rouse people to action and good examples of this are the stirring freedom songs of the black people of South Africa and the Civil Rights protest movement in the United States. People can be heard in the streets singing the jingles from television and radio advertising.

One of the examples of popular media given in the introduction to this chapter was the calypso songs of the Caribbean. The calypso below was sung and composed in the local English dialect by 'The Mighty Sheller', a leading calypso singer in the island of St Vincent in the early 1970s.

They say ninety thousand, is our population.
One hundred and fifty square miles of land,
For we to live on.
One-fifth of the population is strong and healthy women.
Don't doubt everyone of them could produce children.

Chorus: There is a need I see, in this country,
           So start plan your family.
           Otherwise is more delinquency.
           More crime and poverty.
           So do some family planning, and help the situation.
           Join St Vincent Planned Parenthood Association.

136

Young men of this country I want you to realise
If you join in this exercise, you can get yourself sterilise
Come take the operation, it's simple and quite easy
That wouldn't prevent you from enjoying sexual activity.

Our local association will give you some good advice
When you need it come and visit. The staff is helpful and nice
So my fellow Vincentian, I am telling you in advance
I feel family planning is of national importance.

The Ladin Gabas project in Nigeria that was described earlier in the chapter also uses songs. The song leader sings the story, while the others join in the chorus after each verse. The song below is one they developed to tell about the symptoms, cause, prevention and treatment of malaria.

Chorus: Good health we want.
          Let's all be healthy.

Verses: Fever is bothering me,
          Mosquitos bring it.
          Standing water around out house
          causes mosquitoes to breed.
          Let us take the children to the clinic.
          That they may stay well.
          We take them to the clinic for Daraprim.
          That they may stay well.
          Broken pots and tin pans.
          Let us bury them.

In a nutrition project in Uganda, a popular ballad singer was asked to compose a song about kwashiorkor and its prevention. The song he prepared, called 'Kitobero', was made available as a record and was a great success. Songs have been used in education of the public on AIDS in many countries and are particularly valuable in reaching young people. One project in Zaire recorded songs about AIDS and installed cassette recorders on public buses to play the songs to the passengers.

Songs were also an important part of a health education programme directed at young people aged 13–18 years in 11 countries including Mexico, Peru and Bolivia. The message, 'It's OK to say no' was the theme of the campaign that was directed at reducing the incidence of teenage pregnancies. Following initial research, it was found that the most important interest of the young people was music and the project produced two songs, one on each side of a record, with a colour record jacket which opened into an attractive poster.

Focus group discussions (see Chapter 11 for more detail on this research method) were carried out. These established the acceptability of the following points: (1) young people, both men and women, should be sexually responsible for their own actions; (2) it's OK to say no; (3) young people can go to specific identified places for professional counselling or guidance; and (4) positive role models, i.e. persons they look up to, are helpful to young people who want to be responsible.

The singers were carefully chosen to appeal to the young people, who accepted the main messages in their own lives. Tatiana, a young Mexican woman, and Johnny, a young Puerto Rican man, were selected. A competition was held with more than 20 professional composers participating to select five songs which would be popular. The final choice of two, selected by pre-testing with groups of

Fig. 7.4 Tatiana and Johnny

young people, were: 'When we are together' and 'Wait'. These were marketed like commercial songs with the usual promotional material to accompany them.

The words for one of their songs were:

(She)	There's no need to run, there is no need to run.
	Love that is rushed, Is love that is lost.
(Chorus)	Understand!
(Both)	Let's not love at the wrong time.
(Chorus)	Stop!

The songs reached the top of the hit parade in Mexico within six weeks of their release. Not only were the songs heard by millions of young people, but they even made a profit that could be spent on further projects for young people. Patrick Coleman, from the Population Communication Services of Johns Hopkins University who managed this exciting and innovative programme, draws the following lessons from their experience:

- Choose the most appropriate medium to reach the intended audience – in this case, popular music.

138

- Involve professionals who are experienced in the chosen medium and make sure they are the best available.
- Develop a high-quality product that will attract the commercial sector. Commercial support for a social message helps to meet production expenses, assures wider spread of the message, and may even generate income for programme expansion.
- Use a medium which has a big regional and national audience. This enables a large-scale project to draw on resources not readily available to a local organization working alone and brings additional attention to the project because of its international scope.

Working on this large scale needs considerable initial funding and may not be possible for you. But it should still be possible for you to use music and songs in your community. The principle of involving local musicians and maintaining a high standard of entertainment also applies – even for community-based projects.

Songs can be used to promote community participation and challenge social injustice. A programme working in the Dominican Republic started a Nutrition Education and Recuperation Centre in a poor section of the provincial capital, Barahona. Meetings were held with the women who discussed family planning and sex, prevention of disease, and the promotion of good health in low-income communities. The women made wall-posters with cuttings from newspapers and magazines, composed and learned songs and carried out some drama on a social issue. The songs they sing deal with social issues.

Let me tell you, my friend,
These days we can't cope.
Rice costs 34 cents,
And it's 40 cents for soap.

In the neglected slums,
We're tired of having to say:
Light costs too much
And we can't afford to pay.

Chorus: Onward, women, onward!
         Together we must strive,
         Let us unite
         To better our lives.

Visual art

Another form of popular media that can be used in health education is visual art. Magazines and newspapers are often dominated by 'commercial art' which is often based on Western pictures. However, most cultures have traditional forms of visual art. In societies where the level of literacy is low, pictures often have a specific purpose of telling stories. Examples of this are the religious paintings and stained-glass windows of early Christian Europe and temple-carvings and religious wall-paintings of India. These traditional visual art-forms show themselves in many ways; from the decorations on houses, religious buildings, temples, trucks and public buildings; carvings in wood and stone; designs on fabrics and clothes; and posters, paintings and calendars.

In Ghana there are traditional symbols that have quite specific meanings. One symbol, 'Sankofa', means combining traditional with modern and was used as the title of a WHO film describing a primary health programme in Ghana.

Fig. 7.5 Ghana Ashanti symbols

In Sri Lanka the accelerated national immunization adopted a symbol based on the traditional *pachayudhya* symbol used from ancient times to ward off evil and disease especially in children. The trident, chank, sword, bow and arrow and amulets are symbols to conquer disease and malevolent spirits.

There are many examples of the use of folk art and design in health education communication.

Fig. 7.6 Sri Lanka immunization sticker with traditional 'pachayudhya' symbol

INYANDZA LEYO
MASWATI

ASILWE NE AIDS!

Fig. 7.7 Swaziland AIDS leaflet with traditional design

Other popular media

Once we start looking carefully we can uncover other forms of popular communication that could be used in health education. In many streets and markets there are street merchants selling goods, including medicines, charms and traditional ointments. There might be fortune tellers and street entertainers. Listen to them and you can learn a great deal from the methods they use to attract interest and persuade people to buy their products.

In the towns of Nepal there are fortune-tellers who tell the future from cards. A health education project assisted by UNICEF produced an additional card that contained a goddess on one side and a diagram promoting oral rehydration solution on the other.

Fig. 7.8 Fortune-telling card promoting oral rehydration therapy in Nepal

Some problems in using popular media

Two examples will be given of the problems of using popular media. In the small mountain country of Lesotho in Southern Africa the *pitso* is a traditional gathering where the chief consults the community, and matters of importance are discussed. Many development agencies recognize the value of this traditional meeting place and hold *pitsos* to announce a range of practices in health and other areas. Some people feel that with the increasing number of *pitsos*, this traditional form of communication has been spoilt by the development agencies and lost its meaning to the community.

The Family Planning Council of Nigeria and the International Planned Parenthood Association collaborated in 1971 to use the Yoruba traditional travelling theatre 'opera' form as a basis for a film for family planning motivation. A well-known and respected actor, Kola Ogunmola, leader of a troupe of travelling players, was asked to participate. Ogunmola was involved in production of the final script and the play was filmed in a Yoruba village with his company playing the main roles and local people as extras.

The story centred on the dilemma facing a forward-looking urban family who planned their family. They returned to their village for a wedding and saw the difficulties their brother faced in providing for his large family. The rural brother asked the town-dwelling brother to take one of his sons with him and look after him, and a disagreement arose. The new bride was taken aside and instructed about the value of family planning. The film, *My Brother's Children*, was produced in Yoruba and English and shown widely in family planning branches, health centres, clinics and hospitals. Twenty thousand copies of a comic strip featuring the same story were also distributed. Showing of the film was followed by discussions by the health workers.

Despite all the careful preparations, the programme is generally considered to have been a failure. A detailed evaluation was undertaken by researchers at Ibadan University which identified some reasons for the film's lack of success. The evaluation showed that, although understood and enjoyed by health and family planning workers, it had less impact on the community for which it was intended. The rural audience did not have much experience of films so the novelty of the filmshow and projector distracted them from the content; the film, lasting almost an hour, contained too much.

The film had been pre-tested with health workers, not the community, so the content did not fit into the local culture – for example, in one scene the family elder gave the bride, not only his blessing, but advice on her future role. This was seen by the community as inappropriate behaviour. The messages of the film mainly reflected the ideas and thought processes of the health and family planning workers rather than how the community saw family planning and their needs. In fact, the character the audience identified with, and felt sympathy for, was not the progressive brother using family planning but the brother living in the village with his large family!

My Brother's Keeper gives us important lessons and reinforces the points made in other chapters in this book – especially understanding behaviour. The impact of popular media is stronger with a live audience compared with the same performance on film – especially if film is an unfamiliar medium. Even if you are using popular artists who are close to the culture of the community, you will need to pre-test your messages with members of the intended audience. Better still, you should involve the community in choosing the messages and ideas to put across in the drama. Perhaps the most important lesson, however, is that it is not enough

Fig. 7.9 Extract from cartoon storybook accompanying Nigerian film *My Brother's Children*

to use an entertaining medium to promote change. If the ideas and practices you are trying to promote are radically different and incompatible to what the community is now practising, and require accompanying economic and social changes, you probably won't succeed!

Ross Kidd and Martin Byram, in their extensive writings on their experiences in the Laedza Batanani theatre programme in Botswana, strongly advocate the use of popular theatre for creating critical consciousness. However, they have also expressed concern about people who try to 'hijack' popular theatre for development purposes. Theatre can become a form of 'top-down' communication which 'packages' health messages in a popular and entertaining form but, in the absence of audience participation, is not so different from mass media. They suggest that we should apply the following questions to theatre activities:

- Whose side is the programme on – the elites or the oppressed?
- Who sets the goals and controls the programmes?
- What are the underlying assumptions about the causes of the problems on which the programme is based? (Does it emphasize 'victim blaming' and individual

143

responsibility or factors at the individual and national level and the role of society?)
- What is the educational method involved in the programme – one-way communication or a genuine two-way dialogue?
- What is the effect of the programme – conditioning people to accept their situation or challenging them to think critically and creatively and discover how to participate in the transformation of their world?

Summary

Look out for folk and popular media in your own community and see if you can mobilize them for health education. Folk media have enormous potential for health education and health promotion. In using popular media you should consider the following:

1. You can brief the artists, actors and musicians, but let them put the health topics in their own words.
2. Any health education carried out through folk media should be based on some initial research on what the community knows, feels and believes about the topic. Pre-test any folk media with a sample of the intended audience before you use it.
3. Involving communities themselves in putting together a drama can be a powerful stimulus for developing community awareness and raising consciousness. It also makes sure that the ideas presented are meaningful and relevant and are more likely to be understood and acted on.
4. You will have more impact by performing live in front of the audience, especially if there is an opportunity for discussion and dialogue between actors and audience. However well-planned and properly tested, folk media can still have a valuable impact when broadcast through mass media such as film, television and radio and played on audio and videocassettes.
5. In using folk media for health avoid moralizing and preaching. Do not destroy their essential characteristics: their popular nature; their entertainment value and ability to deal with social issues.

8. Using media

More and more people in the world have access to some form of mass media such as television, newspapers and radio. In Chapter 2 mass media were compared with other approaches. Mass media are often poorly used to promote one-way 'top-down' communication. However, it is possible to make effective use of media for the promotion of health by applying the guidelines described in earlier chapters, including understanding the audience, pre-testing the message and evaluating impact. This chapter will build on these earlier chapters and:

1. Look at ways in which you can use radio, television and newspapers to communicate health.
2. Give guidelines on how you can produce your own media programmes.
3. Suggest ways of influencing the media to give publicity to your health education and health promotion work.
4. Describe ways in which you can use the media as a resource in your contacts with the community.

Media can seem expensive, difficult to use and to require special skills. Not surprisingly, many people feel powerless to use media. In this chapter I will also look at simple ways you can use the media by getting journalists to report on your activities.

The media revolution

The 1990s are a decade of intense social change. One of the most important factors contributing to this change will be the increase in the numbers of people with some form of access to media. Many problems of visual literacy and unfamiliarity with the conventions of films, television and pictures will disappear as more and more people become exposed to different kinds of media.

Radio is the media channel that now reaches the widest audience. The world is rapidly reaching a situation where most people will have access to a radio either in their family or in their community. There can be problems of supply of batteries, distance from transmitters and poor reception in mountain terrain. Many countries still depend on centralized production of broadcast programmes. However, local radio stations that produce programmes in regional languages and with locally-relevant content are increasingly common.

There are an estimated 960 million television receivers in the world – one for every five persons. Most of these are in the industrialized countries, with one TV for every two persons. But the numbers are rapidly increasing in the developing countries – especially the cities, towns and nearby rural populations. In the 1980s the number of televisions in the developing countries doubled to 350 million – one for every 12 persons, with the highest TV ownership in Asia, Latin America and the Caribbean. The problem of the short range of television transmission is increasingly being overcome with the development of satellites.

In the industrialized countries, the expansion of television has led to a fall in people going to see films in cinemas. However, the filmgoing audience in many developing countries is still large and increasing, especially in Asia. In some countries, though, there has been a shift in filmgoing with people viewing films not at movie houses, but on video.

Video-cassette recorders (VCR) enable audiences to view programmes, even if they are outside the range of TV broadcasts. VCRs are cheaper and break down less often than film projectors. In Asia there is now one VCR for every seven TVs. In some countries such as Ghana and India you can go to a 'video parlour' and pay a fee to watch a video film rather like going to a cinema. VCRs can be fitted to buses. In India more than 12 000 VCRs have been fitted to long-distance buses that travel between states. Some development projects have equipped mobile video units to show video programmes to rural areas. Many countries have shops where you can hire videos.

As literacy and education increase, so does the potential of print media such as newspapers, books and magazines. More magazines are being published, covering a wide range of special interests including football, music, news events, health and films.

Another type of media used by commercial advertisers and health educators are posters that can range in size from quite small to large 'billboards'.

How effective are mass media?

In Chapter 3, the effectiveness of mass media was compared with face-to-face communication. Mass media messages tend to be general and are not always relevant to needs of individual communities. It is also difficult to be selective and target one age-group. And, unlike face-to-face approaches, there is no direct feedback. However, if carried out well, mass media has the advantage of being able to reach a large audience rapidly – and does not require an infrastructure of fieldworkers. Although many people prefer face-to-face communication, lack of time, shortage of fieldworkers and difficulties of transport can make mass media the only realistic way of working.

Mass media are sometimes used poorly with a lack of audience research, dull programmes and inappropriate messages. In fact, well-planned mass media health education can achieve a great deal:

- *Behaviour change* – when the behaviour is a 'one-time' behaviour such as attending an immunization clinic, simple to perform or the community is favourably disposed to implement it and is merely requiring a trigger for action.
- *Agenda setting* – bringing an issue to the public's attention so that they begin talking about it and raising it at meetings.
- *Creating a favourable climate of knowledge and opinion* – media can provide specific knowledge about issues that will influence felt needs of communities; they can provide a favourable background for community-based programmes and health education activities at clinics.
- *Telling people about new ideas* – media can make people aware of new discoveries or 'innovations' such as oral rehydration. Whether people will actually act on this information depends on the idea, its complexity and whether it meets a perceived need in the community.

Who uses media?

You have already seen that, in order for a communication to be effective, it must be specific to the intended audience. Different media reach different groups in the community: people who are not literate will not read newspapers; television may only be watched by people in towns – and only by those who have the money to afford it; and programmes broadcast in the daytime will not reach those at work.

So it is important to find out if your intended audience watch television, listen to the radio or read newspapers or magazines. If they do, find out *when* they watch and *which* programmes they like. This information may already be available. It is common for newspapers, radio and television stations to carry out research on the size and characteristics of their audiences and readers. Try to find out if audience surveys have been carried out and if the results are available.

Audience surveys may not be available, so look for opportunities to find out which media your intended audience uses and likes. An example of this was the AIDS Control Programme in Swaziland which carried out a survey of youth to find out which radio programmes young people listened to. This information was used to design radio programmes that would reach as many young people as possible.

Decisions on advice to be presented on media

The concepts introduced in earlier chapters on the influences on health, understanding behaviour and communication all need to be taken into account when considering what information to include in media. As you can see in Figure 3.6, advice should be epidemiologically correct, realistic, acceptable and easy to understand. As you do not have the chance to obtain direct feedback from an audience you should always carefully pre-test the message, words, pictures and ideas to make sure that they are clear, relevant and acceptable.

Choice of formats

In the past, formats used by health educators have been mainly advertisements, spot announcements and health talks. The public can regard advertisements as a nuisance which interrupts favourite programmes. It can be a time for leaving the room to go to the toilet or putting on the kettle for a cup of tea! Many people develop resistance to the obvious sales pressure of commercial advertising and persuasive messages used in health education. However, there are many other ways to present information on health in ways that are both entertaining and effective. Success has been achieved using interviews, dramas, popular music, and stories that use traditional and cultural forms. I have listed some of these different formats below. An outline of a typical magazine format is given on page 150. Which formats do you think might be the best ones for communicating your health messages?

In Anambra State, Nigeria, 43 mini-dramas on family planning were used in the popular variety show *In a Lighter Mood*. During this period attendance at the major clinic in Enugu increased from 50 clients a month to more than 120. After the first month, an average of 45 per cent of clients mentioned the show as their source of referral. In a survey carried out in the streets, more than half the sample had watched the programme the night before. More than two-thirds of those could give the address of the clinic mentioned.

In India a soap opera was produced, called *Hum Log* (meaning 'Our People') that used stories about ordinary people to promote ideas of equal status for women, family harmony and small family-sizes. An average of 50 million people watched each of 156 episodes during 17 months during 1984/5. It was evaluated

147

through a survey of 1170 viewers and analysis of 500 letters received from viewers. Evaluation showed that the first twelve programmes were not as popular as later ones. The earlier programmes put too much emphasis on family-planning messages and not enough on entertainment and establishing the characters for the drama.

In Swaziland a six-month radio campaign was run to promote home-made oral rehydration solution. Twenty radio programmes of 15 minutes each, 46 radio inserts of 5 minutes length each and 22 spot announcements were developed. A leaflet with mixing instructions was produced and posters were displayed at health clinics. Training workshops were held for health workers and participants then trained other volunteer helpers. Local volunteers were given yellow flags to hang outside their homes to show that they could help with treatment of diarrhoea. Evaluation of the campaign showed that 85 per cent of the country's population had been exposed to the campaign. A survey before the campaign showed that only 15 per cent could correctly make up the solution. After the campaign this increased to 42 per cent.

Formats in newspapers and magazines

News. Descriptions of recent events often accompanied by photographs.

Future events. Details of future events, public announcements.

Advertisements. These can be any size from 'small ads' up to full-pages advertising commercial products and even containing health messages.

Features. Features are longer articles describing events or reviewing topics. They do not necessarily deal with news events and can contain items of general interest, short stories, science topics, advice for readers on finance. Health is often a subject for features such as descriptions of a new disease, problems of rural communities, etc.

Letters. These are usually sections with letters from the public responding to various issues. The letters section is popular so it is a good idea to send in your letters on health topics.

Special interest sections, including: women's page, food section, finance, sports page; often these contain an 'advice column' responding to issues raised by listeners that can include health or even relationships with other persons.

Formats on radio and television

News. On most radio and television stations news bulletins are an important part of the daily output. If it is a local radio station, local news will also be included. To have your health education activity mentioned in a news bulletin is highly desirable because it gives it widespread coverage, credibility and importance and does not cost you anything.

Spot announcements. These can be public service announcements, such as when clinics are open, immunization programmes and availability of casualty services. These will usually be broadcast free. On commercial stations it is also possible to 'buy time' in the form of commercials. This could be useful for a campaign.

Slogans and jingles. Slogans are catchy short sentences, designed to attract attention, usually based on well-known sayings or rhymes. They can identify a campaign. Jingles are slogans set to music and can make a slogan more memorable, be used to identify a programme, person, radio station or theme.

Discussions. There are many kinds of discussion programmes. The one most commonly used on radio is the 'group' or 'round-table' discussion. A group of people of different opinions and from possible different backgrounds discuss a common subject under the guidance of a chairman.

'Phone-in' programmes. Programmes in which listeners ring in to the studio either 'live' or 'off air' and give their views, ask questions or ask for advice. Their calls are dealt with either by the broadcaster along with, or by an expert in the studio or by a panel involved in discussion.

Interview. A discussion in question-and-answer form between the broadcaster and one (or two) guests. The interview can also be used to find out opinions of the 'man in the street' either in a studio situation or outside in the community (when it is then called 'vox pop').

Talks and documentaries. Five-to-fifteen minute talks by one person are occasionally used but, unless the broadcaster is very skilled, can be boring. Documentaries explore a single topic and include different effects, e.g. drama, music, interview, storytelling, descriptions, sound effects.

Drama. Long or short plays, 'soap opera', comedy sketches, serials, drama/documentaries. 'Soap opera' is the name for a weekly or even daily drama series using the same characters, such as the American soap opera *Dallas*. As discussed in Chapter 7, drama has enormous potential for health education because the audience can identify with the characters and their problems. Soap operas are even more powerful because the characters can become like family friends.

Music. This is an essential part of broadcasting, whether it is traditional music, or popular local music, musical jingles or background music to programmes. Music will attract people to watch and listen and spot announcements, public service messages and slogans can be inserted in music programmes. Jingles or songs with a message can become very popular and people will sing them and remember the message.

149

Quizzes and panel games. Quizzes with panels of guests are popular and most people watching or listening try to answer the questions themselves and learn something from the answers. Sometimes listeners have to write in with a correct answer for a prize. This gives feedback on how many people heard the programme and understood the message.

Magazine programmes. This popular format combines different short elements: music, drama, stories, sketches, interviews, comedy, discussion. They are linked by a presenter and are sometimes aimed at a particular audience such as women or farmers. An example of a typical magazine programme is given below.

Example of typical 30-minute magazine programme and how it could be used in social development

---

Music:	Theme music
Announcer:	Introduction and highlights
	music
	Soap opera episode or drama
	music
Announcer:	Link with announcement about theme of programme
	Story or interview or local feature
	Talk by expert related to theme, or by announcer
	music
Announcer:	Quiz related to theme of programme
	music
Announcer:	Answers and conclusion
Music:	Theme music

Social marketing – can health be sold as a product?

Social marketing is the name given to the approach of applying commercial advertising methods to promoting healthy behaviours. Social marketers place emphasis on the 'four P's': product, price, place and promotion.

- *Product* – the suggested action/behaviour change must be relevant, necessary and presented in an attractive way.
- *Price* – the product must be affordable.
- *Place* – the product must be accessible and available where the people are.
- *Promotion* – effort must be put into telling people about the product, repeating key messages in an attractive way.

Two recent examples where the social marketing approach has been used in many countries are the promotion of condoms and oral rehydration solution (ORS). In both cases, attention was paid to designing packaging and giving suitable names to make them attractive and interesting. Care was also taken to stock local shops with them at affordable prices. They were promoted with songs, jingles, posters and eye-catching campaign symbols called 'logos'. See Figure 3.15 for a social marketing strategy for ORS in Honduras.

Fig. 8.1 This logo, used in Egyptian packets of oral rehydration salts, was adopted after pre-testing with groups of women in the community

Can the methods for promoting commercial products be used to promote health? It is easy to see how these methods can be used for some health practices such as condoms, oral rehydration packages, latrines, seat belts and special weaning foods. It is not so easy to see the method applied to other health behaviours, such as keeping to one faithful partner or spacing one's children.

But, even if we cannot apply commercial advertising on the scale of large companies, there are important lessons that we can apply: researching the target audiences, ensuring that the desired practice is relevant, affordable and easy to carry out; making sure that programmes are attractive, well-presented and pre-tested; being aware of the importance of evaluating the impact and using the results of evaluations for future planning.

Influencing the media

You may not be in a position to prepare radio or television programmes, and feel that much of what is described above is not relevant to your situation. However, making your own programmes is only one of many different ways of using media. Indeed, it can be easier, cheaper and more effective to encourage newspapers, radio and television to take up health issues in their general news and programme content.

It is worthwhile finding out the names of the journalists and writers who put together programmes on television and radio and write for local newspapers and magazines. They will usually be looking out for interesting stories. You can meet informally and tell them about some of the health issues you are involved in, and:

- suggest some health topics that could be included in a drama they are preparing – for example one of the characters might develop a health problem and receive advice from another person;
- provide background papers on health topics and copies of any leaflets. Make yourself available if they need someone to interview;
- provide questions on health topics that could be included in a quiz programme;
- write letters responding to topics covered in the newspaper or current affairs that they can put in their letters page.

You may feel that what you are doing is worthwhile and important. However, in order for it to receive media coverage two conditions will have to be fulfilled: *your activity has to be something that the media will see as 'newsworthy'*; and *you have to tell the media what is happening*.

Newspapers, television and radio are always looking out for something interesting to report. They keep a diary of local events and decide which are sufficiently interesting to make it worth sending a reporter to cover the event. But they are usually very busy so will only be attracted if the topic is:

- of *interest* to the community – a programme to deal with a serious disease, a visit by a famous person, activities by local leaders;
- *topical* and relevant to other issues in the news;
- *unusual*, strange;
- anything *new* such as the launching of a new campaign; or
- a *scandal* or controversial topics such as commercial companies promoting dangerous products.

You should look out for activities in your health education programmes that might be of interest to the media. You can even deliberately include 'media events' into your programme to attract the press. Some examples of what can be done are: a ceremony with invited guests to launch a new campaign; a celebration with invited guests to mark an anniversary – the first year of the immunization programme, the hundredth latrine to be completed, the thousandth child to receive measles immunization; an exhibition with an official opening ceremony; an announcement of a 'new discovery'; and a presentation of prizes for a competition.

Look for opportunities for making your media events even more interesting. One approach is to invite well-known people as guests. For example, in Lesotho the Ministry of Health invited their King to launch their immunization programme and be photographed giving oral polio vaccine to a baby.

You should also look for ways of making it *visually interesting* so that newspapers will want to include a photograph. People can be dressed in costumes, there can be a procession carrying a coffin with the number of children who have died of the disease, a latrine can be carried on the back of a truck through the town.

As part of your media event, you could set up a *press conference* which is a meeting where journalists can ask questions and find out information. It is always a good idea to put important information on a sheet of paper as reporters can easily make mistakes in reporting technical information. The best way to let the media know what you are doing is by preparing a *'press release'* (see Figure 8.2). This is a written document of not more than one page in length, neatly typed with an attention-getting headline. It should provide information on what you are doing by answering these questions:

- *WHAT will be happening?* Describe the event. Give names of important people participating and details of activities that might make a good photograph.
- *WHY will it take place?* Give background details; explain why the activity is taking place. Supply some facts and figures that they can quote in a story – e.g. how many children died of pneumonia last year in that community.
- *WHERE will it take place?* Give precise details of how to get there.
- *WHEN* will it take place? Give the date and time of day.

In addition to background information on the topic the press release should also give an address and telephone number of someone to contact if they need further information.

On December 1st, World AIDS Day, a procession of floats and marching bands will begin at the City Hall at 10 a.m. and proceed through Main Street to City Square. They will then be addressed by a group of community leaders including the Mayor, the Chief Medical Officer, the captain of the national football team, the Minister for Woman's Affairs and the Archbishop. The highlight of the festival will be the release of 8000 balloons, one for each person who has died of AIDS this year. That night at 8 p.m. a candle-light vigil will be held at the Cathedral and Grand Mosque.

Background information: 8000 people have died of AIDS in our country so far. Surveys have shown that between 5 and 10 per cent of the public are carriers of the AIDS virus – healthy but capable of infecting others. Already 200 babies have died of AIDS this year. There is no cure or vaccine for AIDS so the emphasis must be on prevention. Everyone should be encouraged to:

- keep to one regular sexual partner;
- avoid having sex with others whom you suspect have multiple partners or go to prostitutes;
- when in doubt about your sexual partner use a condom during intercourse;
- report to your nearest clinic for treatment if you think you have a sexually transmitted disease.

For further information:
James Munyango, Coordinator World AIDS Day Celebrations tel. 54380
Joy Kalemaro, Publicity coordinator, AIDS Forum tel. 54620

Fig. 8.2 A sample press release

Before you issue the press release there are some points to consider: are you allowed by your employers to contact the press and make statements to press or radio? Will you need clearance? If you are not allowed, is there someone who can be asked to speak on your behalf? Are you sure that the information you are providing is both technically correct and fits in with national policy?

It is likely that a reporter will want to interview you for further information. You might be asked to give an interview on radio or television. This will give a valuable opportunity to get key points across but you must be well prepared! Discuss in advance the questions that will be asked. Do not be afraid to suggest additional questions the interviewer may not have thought of. Some tips to help you give an effective interview are presented in the table.

Tips for being interviewed on radio and television

1. Be prepared – know your facts and figures or have details handy.
2. Be clear and concise; keep to the point. If time is limited make sure that you get the most important points across first; why it is important, who is affected and what people can do about it.
3. Make it interesting! Sound enthusiastic. Have notes to refer to but try to avoid reading them out, as this will sound boring. Build in personal examples, human stories (but be careful of giving names and breaching confidentiality).
4. Keep the language simple and avoid technical words. Give statistics in ways people will find it easy to grasp (rather than saying 15 per cent of children die in the first year, try saying 'one in six children die' or 'every hour a baby dies of malnutrition').

5. Make it clear when you are speaking on behalf of an organization and when you are giving your own views.
6. Keep calm! If you don't like a question, don't refuse to answer but take a lesson from politicians by changing the subject or asking a question back!
7. If the interview is being broadcast 'live' be careful what you say. If it is being recorded, don't be afraid to ask to repeat part of the interview.

Combining mass media with face-to-face education

Mass media will have more impact when combined with face-to-face communication. When people listen to radio programmes or read newspapers they usually discuss the content with others in their family or community. This natural process can be built upon in your health education programme. For example, you can brief your fieldworkers in advance to follow up broadcasts with discussions with the community in clinics, on home visits or at meetings.

People often listen to radio in groups. You can deliberately encourage this by setting up a *radio listening group* – or 'radio forum' – of between 10 and 20 people who may either be an existing group in the community or one specially set up, such as a group of mothers at a health centre. A group leader introduces the programme and, after listening to the programme, a discussion is held on the content. Experience with radio listening groups suggest the following guidelines.

Fig. 8.3 Radio learning group in Haryana State, India

1. prepare the meeting place and study materials

2. welcome the members

3. turn on the radio

4. refer to the flipchart pictures

5. turn off the radio

6. read the study guide

7. discuss each question

8. fill in the report form

9. agree on individual or collective action

10. close the meeting

Fig. 8.4 Organizing radio listening groups in Botswana

- Use visual aids such as posters or a flip chart to help the discussion. They can be shown to the group during the radio programme to emphasize key points, add a visual dimension and assist the discussion at the end. Provide leaflets for the audience to take away.
- Ask the group questions to make them think about the programme and the key messages. Note their comments and send them back to the programme organizers. This provides valuable feedback on the relevance of the programme and the needs of the communities.
- Mobilize other workers in the community to help you. School teachers and fieldworkers from health, agriculture, family-planning and literacy services could lead the listening groups. You can provide simple training to introduce the health topics, use the visual aids and simple group discussion skills.

A well-known example of the use of the use of the radio forum is the *Mtu ni afya* campaign that took place in 1973 in Tanzania. In this campaign twelve 30-minute radio programmes were each broadcast twice a week over a twelve-week period. Through an intensive programme of seminars, 75 000 study-group leaders were trained and an estimated 2 million participants listened to the broadcasts in study groups. A manual was produced for the group leaders, study guides for the participants and a series of flip charts to be used during the broadcasts. The first ten minutes of each radio programme consisted of an introductory signature tune, news about the progress of the campaign and songs and poems. A study of health practices before and after the campaign showed some limited changes in health practices, including use of latrines.

Botswana is another African country that has used radio forums. Figure 8.4 is taken from their excellent handbook on designing radio forums. Even if you cannot produce your own radio programmes you can still use this approach in your community. Any health broadcast provides an opportunity for a group to meet. If there is a regular broadcast on health you can arrange for a group to meet and listen to it. You can write and find out in advance the topics to be covered and prepare suitable discussion questions.

Audio-cassettes

One disadvantage of radio is that the time of broadcast may not be very convenient for the group. This problem is easily overcome by recording the programme on a cassette recorder so the group can listen to it at a time that suits everyone. Audio-cassette recorders are becoming increasingly common and have many advantages:

- You are not restricted to a particular broadcast time.
- Broadcast programmes can be used repeatedly with many groups (but be careful of copyright laws).
- You can stop the cassette during the programme, repeat sections and discuss points when they arise.

Radio suffers from the disadvantage that programmes are directed at the general population and do not meet the specific needs of local groups. However it is not difficult to record locally-relevant health education programmes on cassettes. These can be played to local audiences while waiting at clinics, to groups of women in workshops and other locations.

A well-known example of this was a health education project in Guatemala carried out by Colle and co-workers. They carried out a small research study on the lifestyle and needs of the women in the community. This study identified

Fig. 8.5 An audiocassette

their concerns and present practices and showed that most women spent some time in the week at a public laundry facility. They recorded a health education programme which used an entertaining magazine format which included drama, music and talks. Members of the community were paid to play the cassettes at the public washing-places and change the cassettes regularly. A different programme was prepared for each day during a three-week period. An evaluation of the impact of the programme showed improvements both in knowledge and adoption of health practices.

Practical broadcasting techniques

You do not need sophisticated equipment to produce simple programmes for your own community. But it is worth making your recordings to as high a standard as possible. If they are good enough, radio stations will be prepared to broadcast them to reach a wide audience. The experienced radio broadcaster Maggie Holt has suggested the following advice as well as the 'Tips for being interviewed' on pages 153–4 and the 'Guidelines on good broadcasting' on pages 158–9.

The tape recorder

This is the essential tool of the trade. Portable tape recorders are usually battery-operated. Always test the tape recorder before you take it anywhere – and test it

Fig. 8.6 Reel-to-reel recorder

again before starting to record! After finishing a recording it is always a good idea to play back a few seconds to make sure it has recorded. Take adequate supplies of tapes and batteries. High-quality programmes are usually made on 'reel-to-reel' recorders but good-quality recordings can also be made on cassette recorders that are simpler to operate. The best recorders have controls for sound levels that you can adjust according to the volume of the sound you are recording. However, most ordinary cassette machines have automatic level controls which are easier to use – but cannot produce special effects such as 'fading' music at the end of a programme.

The microphone

The secret to a good recording is to use a microphone. Avoid using the built-in microphones on cassette recorders as they tend to pick up the sound of the machinery of the cassette recorder. Keep the microphone about six inches from the mouth of the person speaking. It is best to have the microphone on a stand. If you do hold it by hand, wrap the cable around your fingers so the cable doesn't make a noise when you move. If you are recording outside, wind can be a problem: try to record in a protected area, such as underneath a coat with your back to the wind. If it is very noisy, turn the recording level down and hold the microphone closer. If a room echoes, turn the recording level down and hold the microphone closer. Try not to move the microphone too much. If recording music, position the microphone nearer the voice(s) than the instrument and hold the microphone further away than for speech. The above are only rough guides. It is always best to try recording a little bit and play back the recording to find out if it sounds right.

Editing

This is the process by which you can remove unwanted parts of a recording such as background noises, unnecessary questions and mistakes and join several different recordings together to make a programme. Tape from a reel-to-reel recording can be edited by cutting the tape and joining together the parts that you want. 'Dub' editing is a simpler process by which you connect two recorders and record the different parts you want from the original recordings on to a 'master' tape.

Guidelines on good broadcasting

---

1. **Be brief**: Assume the listener gets bored easily and can very easily 'switch off' mentally or physically at any time.
2. **Be entertaining**: Above all the listener wants to be entertained by the broadcast; make it as lively and interesting as possible. Try to make the message more acceptable by use of music, comedy or drama. Don't lecture.
3. **Be clear**: It is no use burying the message too far in the entertainment, or making it obscure. Be simple, use straightforward ordinary language (local dialect). In a book it is always possible to read a section again if you do not understand it first time. You can't do this with radio or television so it is a good idea to repeat the message at different times in the programme. Speak clearly and don't rush. Addresses, dates and phone numbers (and any important names or numbers) should always be repeated.

4. **Aim for maximum impact**: Always try to start a programme with something that catches the attention, e.g. baby crying, music, jingle, crash, or a striking word or question. End with something that people will remember.
5. **Dialogue or discussion** is always more interesting than only one person talking. It is very difficult to hold attention with one voice.
6. **Aim for variety**: Don't put in too much speech or too long pieces of music. Try putting a music background to the speech, use different voices, ask questions; keep the listeners guessing what will come next; try not to be predictable.
7. **Choose carefully the people you interview:** When interviewing or choosing participants for discussion programmes *choose your people carefully*. They also must speak clearly and simply and be interesting.
8. **Put 'colour' into interviews**: Create a picture in the mind of your listeners that will help them to set the interview into its situation. Describe your surroundings, the family, the area, what's going on.
9. **Ask 'how' and 'why' questions** that allow people to express ideas and opinions; avoid questions that just need yes or no answers.
10. **Write for the listener or viewer**: Always think of one person the other side of the microphone and address them personally, as you would a friend. Be confidential with them and conversational. Say 'you' and 'we', not 'listeners'. Use the colloquial language of ordinary people.

Print media

Newspapers and magazines can be a useful way of reaching the community with your health education messages. Obviously you will only be able to reach those who can read and can afford to buy them. But that audience will often include opinion leaders and influential persons.

Leaflets

These are the most common way of using print media in health education. The simplest leaflet is a single sheet of paper, printed on both sides, and folded in half or into thirds. Leaflets can be larger with two or more sheets of paper. Once there are more than five sheets it is common to use the term 'booklet'. Leaflets can be a useful reinforcement for individual and group sessions and serve as a reminder of the main points that you have made. Even if people cannot read, they can ask others to read them for them. Leaflets are helpful for sensitive subjects such as sex when people are too shy to ask but can pick up a leaflet and read the information.

Suitable leaflets may already be available for your health education work. However, leaflets produced by others may not be directly relevant, either because of language or content so you may have to produce leaflets for your own community. However, these do not have to be expensively produced to a sophisticated standard – especially if the topic is one that your target readership is interested in.

A useful starting-point is to look at leaflets produced in other programmes in your country or from abroad. This will give you ideas on how you can adapt the ideas to your own situation. Make the language simple with pictures and try out draft versions to make sure that they are understood. Always include an address where people can go for further information. Give them out at talks or counselling sessions, leave them in public places and make them available on demand after a radio or television programme. Think of places in the community

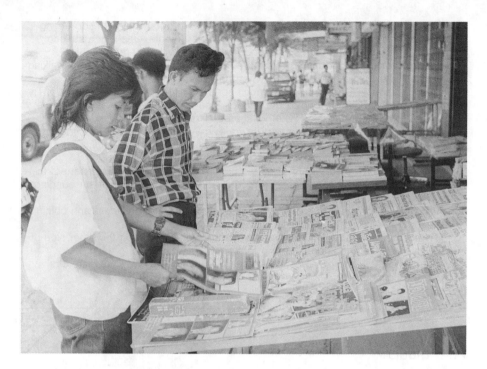

Fig. 8.7 Magazines on sale in Thailand

where you can leave the leaflets and people might come across them. Look out for opportunities to distribute them in different ways such as wage packets, voters' registration forms, electricity bills and rent statements, etc. A simple checklist that you can use for testing out a leaflet is:

- Is it interesting to look at?
- Does it contain relevant information for the target readership?
- Does it avoid distracting irrelevant information?
- Is the language easy to read?
- Does it avoid complicated technical words?
- Is the advice presented realistic and feasible?
- Does it provide the specific information that the target audience actually wants to know?
- Does it tell people where they can get further information?

Magazines

Some health educators have tried producing their own health magazines. For example in India a voluntary organization, the Catholic Hospital Association of India, produces a magazine called *Health Action*. that covers a range of health topics in a visually attractive way and is sold through newspaper outlets. In Zimbabwe, a children's comic called *Action* covers a range of health and environmental issues (see Figure 9.8 in the next chapter). Producing your own magazine is an exciting idea but needs careful thought and preparation. If you plan to give it away through health clinics and schools you will need to obtain funding on a regular basis. The challenge would be to sell it commercially through shops and newspaper stands so that it pays for itself. If people have paid for it they are more

Fig. 8.8 Picture story book on hygiene from Thailand

likely to read and value it than if you simply gave it to them free. However, if you do plan to sell the magazine, it must be well-produced and entertaining so that people are prepared to pay money for it.

In parts of Latin America *photo novelas* are popular. These are storybooks of photographs with accompanying dialogue. In Asia, similar books are widely popular using drawings and text. In Burma a story book was prepared where the theme of leprosy was built into a dramatic story. It was written and drawn by local writers and artists and the finished book was sold alongside other storybooks and widely distributed. In Thailand a storybook on hygiene has been produced.

Producing your own magazine is a big task. You may not have the time or resources to take this on – then it would be better to try to interest existing magazines in covering health topics. Most of what was discussed above about influencing the media, writing press releases and staging media events is also relevant to magazines. Try to find out who reads the different newspapers and magazines. There may be specialist magazines aimed at reaching young people, businessmen and women that could be suited for your needs.

Some tips on clear writing

Whether you are writing the words for a poster, leaflet, newspaper article, or storybook you will have to pay attention to your writing style. In looking at written materials we usually separate out the following two concepts:

- *Legibility* refers to whether the actual words can be distinguished on the paper; writing which is too faint, too small, uses complicated typefaces or where the ink has smudged are all difficult to read.
- *Readability* refers to how easy it is to understand the meaning of the text: using too many unfamiliar words, long sentences, complicated sentence structures with different sections; long paragraphs, crowded pages and no headings can all make text difficult to understand.

A piece of writing may be clear to you but that does not mean that others will also understand it. Young children may still be developing their reading skills. Your audience may have left school early or have only learnt to read as adults. The written material may even be in the community's second language or be written in a different style. For example, in India a translation was made of the WHO publication *The Primary Health Care Worker* from English into Hindi. An evaluation study showed that the book was not understood because the language used was a formal style using 'polite' expressions rather than everyday language. Many health education writings were originally written in English and you must be careful to translate with appropriate language. This can be difficult as the language may not have local equivalents for technical words. If you have translated something from English it's always a good idea to ask someone else to translate the text back into English and see if it has kept the meaning.

Writing in simple language is not easy. It is worth studying the style used by newspapers, magazines and books that are read by your community. See if you can adopt their language, choice of words and general approach. Each language will have its own rules about writing clearly and simply and some tips on clear writing are given here.

- Write simply; avoid using a 'literary' style.
- Keep sentences short; avoid long sentences with too many sections; vary the length of sentences to keep the writing interesting.
- Use simple words that are understood by the intended audience; avoid abbreviations and technical words; if you use specialized words, make sure you explain them.
- Use active rather than passive forms of verbs: i.e. use 'poor hygiene causes diarrhoea' rather than 'diarrhoea is caused by poor hygiene'.
- Lay the text out on the page to make it easy to read – avoid crowding the page with writing – space it out.
- Use lists and 'bullets' (dots or symbols in front of each point on the line as is done with this list) to bring out main points.
- Avoid small print and fancy typefaces; use headlines, **bold** letters, *italics* to emphasize different sections and important words; keep the use of capital ('upper case') letters to a minimum.
- Use diagrams and pictures to explain ideas; put them close to the part of the text they refer to; make sure that they can be easily understood by the reader.

Posters

Posters can range in size from large billboards to small notices. Production of posters has dominated the work of many health education services. They have been given too much emphasis, compared with more effective approaches such as community mobilization, drama, group teaching and one-to-one. By themselves posters have little value. They are useful mainly to bring a topic to the attention of the community, reinforce a message that the public is receiving through other channels such as radio and face-to-face and provide a talking-point for discussion. Examples of appropriate use include posters:

- used to reinforce the main theme of a radio campaign;
- in a clinic that is used as the theme for a talk;
- put up in a village to draw attention to a community meeting;
- outside a shop to say that condoms are available.

Some of the issues involved in the design and use of posters, including the content, visual perception, and choice of location were discussed in Chapter 3. A good poster should have a very simple message and not try to say too much. Unlike a wallchart, which is a learning aid to accompany a lesson, a poster has to be clear enough to be understood on its own. It should be 'eye-catching' – gaining attention by use of striking pictures, bright colours or interesting content.

Posters should be displayed where your intended audience will pass them and see them. There is no point in just displaying them at clinics where they will only be seen by a small group of people. You will need to use different locations, depending on the intended audience, e.g. young people, men, pregnant women, long-distance drivers, soldiers. Do not leave the same one up for too long as people will become familiar with it and not notice it.

Other print media

Another popular print medium is the calendar which shows the days of the month and also health education messages. If it is attractive, people will hang it up in

Fig. 8.9 Postage stamps on health from Sri Lanka

their home and workplace. The new page every month provides a way of regularly changing the message and matching it to the season.

Postage stamps have been used by many countries, including Tanzania, Bangladesh and Sri Lanka to carry health education messages.

Some conclusions on using mass media

If well-planned, mass media can be an extremely powerful way of promoting health in your community. They can have an impact on their own as well as create a favourable climate of understanding and concern for a topic that fieldworkers can take advantage of in their face-to-face work. Even if you do not have access to facilities and resources for preparing your own programmes, you can still encourage the media to take up health issues. Some characteristics of different media are shown in Figure 8.10.

The 'P' approach in Figure 8.10 is a helpful guide to remembering the steps in preparing media communication. It was developed by the Population Communication Centre at Johns Hopkins University in the United States.

1. **Analysis**
   Review potential audiences
   Assess existing policies and programmes
   Select sponsoring institutions
   Evaluate communication resources
2. **Design**
   Decide on objectives
   Identify audiences
   Develop messages
   Select media
   Plan for face-to-face reinforcement
   Draw up action plan
3. **Development, pre-testing and revision**
   Develop message concepts
   Pre-test with audience
   Complete message and materials
   Pre-test with audience
4. **Implementation**
   Implement action plan
   Monitor outputs
   Measure impact
5. **Review and re-planning**
   Analyze overall impact
   Replan future activities
   Adjust for changing audience needs

Fig. 8.10 Planning media production using the 'P' Approach (Population Communication Services, Johns Hopkins University)

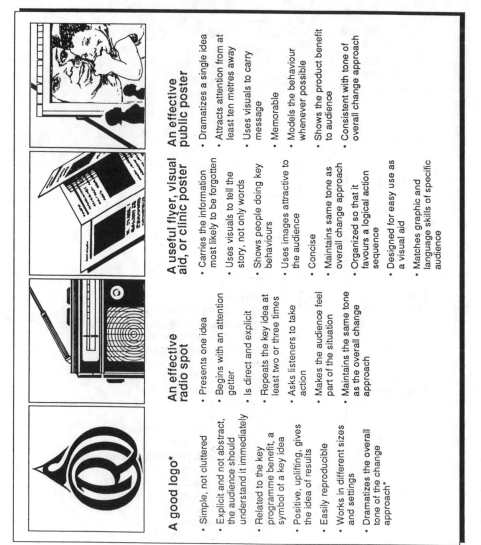

A good logo*

- Simple, not cluttered
- Explicit and not abstract, the audience should understand it immediately
- Related to the key programme benefit, a symbol of a key idea
- Positive, uplifting, gives the idea of results
- Easily reproducible
- Works in different sizes and settings
- Dramatizes the overall tone of the change approach*

An effective radio spot

- Presents one idea
- Begins with an attention getter
- Is direct and explicit
- Repeats the key idea at least two or three times
- Asks listeners to take action
- Makes the audience feel part of the situation
- Maintains the same tone as the overall change approach

A useful flyer, visual aid, or clinic poster

- Carries the information most likely to be forgotten
- Uses visuals to tell the story, not only words
- Shows people doing key behaviours
- Uses images attractive to the audience
- Concise
- Maintains same tone as overall change approach
- Organized so that it favours a logical action sequence
- Designed for easy use as a visual aid
- Matches graphic and language skills of specific audience

An effective public poster

- Dramatizes a single idea
- Attracts attention from at least ten metres away
- Uses visuals to carry message
- Memorable
- Models the behaviour whenever possible
- Shows the product benefit to audience
- Consistent with tone of overall change approach

Fig. 8.11 Characteristics of media

Summary

The following guidelines summarize the main points in this chapter.

1. Decide at the outset what realistically can be achieved by each medium and what cannot. Aim for what can be achieved. Set specific, measurable objectives.
2. Learn lessons from similar campaigns elsewhere and make sure that you do not repeat their mistakes.
3. Base your programme on an analysis of the health issue and its causes. Make sure that the advice you give is accurate, relevant and feasible.
4. Decide which sections of the public you are trying to reach and find out what media they watch, listen to and read. Carry out a simple study on what they believe, feel and know about the health issue. Use this information to make the message specific to the particular audience's needs and to decide on the timing, location and content of your activities.
5. Make friends with journalists and media producers. If you can provide them with interesting stories they will report your activities and provide free publicity.
6. Make your programmes entertaining and avoid 'preaching'. Include popular media such as songs, drama and puppets (see Chapter 7). If you are using dramas and stories, build up the characters and human interest first before including health messages. Wherever possible, involve people with experience in media in producing programmes. Use sources that are trusted by the community.
7. Do not put too many messages into each programme. Always pre-test your programmes and messages with a sample of the target audience before they are broadcast to make sure they are properly understood and accepted.
8. Broadcast programmes as often as possible. Make them available in other formats – distribute the radio programme on audio-cassettes, the TV programme on video, the newspaper article as a leaflet.
9. Try to identify person-to-person advice systems in the community that you could mobilize to reinforce your media activities. Hold discussions with them before the campaign and, if necessary, arrange for some training. Provide written materials to accompany the broadcasts, such as a leaflet.
10. When you use radio or television, prepare reinforcing media such as listening guides, workbooks, simple booklets. A multi-media approach usually will do better than a single channel.
11. Always include a way by which the audience can obtain help or further information, e.g. an address to write to or telephone.
12. Try to build in some mechanism for audience feedback, e.g. letters, and include some method of evaluation. In the short term you should try to find out how many watched, heard or read the programmes and understood the messages. In the longer term you can find out if people remembered the message, accepted the advice and if any change in behaviour took place.

9. Working with children and young people

Almost half the population of most developing countries is made up of children under 15. In carrying out education and communication programmes with children and young people we usually have two broad objectives in mind: the first is to improve the health of the children and young people themselves; the second is to provide the knowledge, attitudes and skills to prepare them for their future lives. This chapter will examine:

1. The special considerations that need to be taken when directing health education at children and young people.
2. How schools can be used to promote the health of young children and future adults.
3. How communication programmes can reach young people out of school.

Special considerations with children and young people

In Chapter 4 you were introduced to the approaches involved in carrying out education and training activities with adults. However, an adult will have fully-developed thinking powers and a wide range of experiences to contribute to the learning. Different approaches are needed – educational programmes for children are different in a number of ways. Children are still *developing*. Depending on his or her age, a child will still be developing his or her understandings of themselves, other people and the world around them.

The period of life between birth and 20 years is one of enormous change. These changes include *physical, intellectual, social and emotional development*. Think about your own experiences with the following groups: children between birth and five years (under-fives or pre-school children), the primary school-aged child (5 to 11), and the older child from 11 to sixteen years. How would you adapt your approach, teaching methods, content and language to each of these groups?

Physical development

Growth in weight and size are the most obvious physical changes. In addition, as children grow they can perform increasingly more complex tasks with their hands and show greater coordination and strength in their movements. From about 10–13 years onwards the sexual organs develop, as do the secondary sexual characteristics of pubic and facial hair and changes in the voice.

Disease, malnutrition and injuries from accidents and violence can affect physical development and lead to reduced growth ('stunting'), deformities and various forms of disability. Good physical development is promoted by a safe environment, adequate diet, preventive health care measures, and opportunities for practising skills involving movement, coordination and handling of objects.

Fig. 9.1 Children

Social, emotional and language development

At birth a baby is dependent on the people around him or her, especially the mother. As a child becomes older he/she interacts with others in the family and through this develop language, beliefs, values, concepts and behaviours that make up the culture of the family, community and society. Important components of social development are the abilities to form relationships, communicate and cooperate with other people. Also important is the development of our ideas about who we are, what we can do, what our future might be. 'Self-concept' is the word used to describe the sum total of our ideas about who we think we are. Our judgement and feelings about whether we feel that we are worthwhile is called 'self-esteem'.

169

This early learning from within the family is called *primary socialization*. Later, a child is subject to influences outside the family, including friends, teachers, books, radio and television and this is called *secondary socialization*. In later childhood and during adolescence, friends – called the 'peer' group – are extremely influential. Anything that affects the stability of the family and relationships with friends can have a damaging effect on social and emotional development. This can include break-up of families from disease, war, family violence, alcohol and influences of poverty and unemployment.

Social and emotional development are promoted by a combination of measures. These include: social and economic measures that give families the resources to maintain their stability and provide a caring environment for their children; advice and help to families on caring for their children; and services providing good-quality care for children separated from their parents for short or longer periods such as pre-school facilities or orphanages.

Intellectual development

Intellectual or 'cognitive' development is concerned with how the growing child develops the ability to *think*. This includes processes of perceiving and building up a mental picture of the surrounding world. It also includes the ability to draw on concepts, rules and procedures to solve problems and make decisions. At the beginning of primary school a child may think in more 'concrete' or specific ways tied to the appearance of things and may only have limited ability for abstract thinking. As a child gets older, he or she develops a greater ability to think in abstract ways, apply concepts, symbols and rules to solve problems. An older child will also have more experiences within and outside the family that can be used to help his or her understanding of the world.

Many factors affect intellectual development. A child has a natural curiosity about the world. The more this curiosity is stimulated with discussions, questions and activities as well as experiences such as visits to interesting places, the more the child's intellect will be developed. Malnutrition and illness have a harmful effect on the way children learn. A hungry child will be tired, inactive and find it difficult to concentrate. Serious malnutrition can lead to permanent disabilities such as blindness and stunting of growth. Illnesses also prevent children from attending school and affect their ability to concentrate and learn. Disabilities such as poor hearing, eyesight and physical movement also affect a child's ability to learn.

Because of the various influences on intellectual development described above, it is not surprising that poverty, poor living conditions and large family size can all have a harmful influence on development. But encouragement of intellectual development of children is not just a matter of meeting needs for food, housing and health care. These physical needs should be supplemented by providing a stimulating and challenging environment. Learning opportunities in the family, community, pre-school and in the school environment can all help a child to achieve his or her potential.

Adolescence

In recent years concern about drugs, alcohol, solvent abuse, smoking and teenage pregnancies has led to greater attention on the period of adolescence. Adolescence involves the following changes:

- *biological changes*: body size and proportions;
- *development of sexuality*, both physical and emotional; sexual organs and secondary sexual characteristics such as hair, breasts;
- *development of ideas about one's identity and future roles*, with possible conflict with expectations of one's family and community.

A biological approach would define adolescence as the time when the human being acquires the ability to reproduce. Another approach is to view adolescence as the period of transition between being a child and acquiring adult status. In traditional societies the period of childhood can be quite short and even quite young children have responsibilities, working in the home and in agriculture. Special ceremonies of initiation often mark the point when the child becomes the adult. These ceremonies publicly recognise that the child has become an adult and often include practical instruction on adult behaviour and sex education.

In Western industrialized societies the period of transition to adult roles is later. During the period up to 16 years a young person is still considered a child, is not allowed to carry out adult work and still attends school. Teenage pregnancy can lead to leaving school early and preventing opportunities for further education. For most children the period of adolescence passes without any problems. For some, it can be a difficult stage – of 'storm and stress' – with conflict, rebellion and disagreements with parents and teachers. This conflict can show itself in experimentation with sex, drugs, smoking and alcohol.

Most developing countries are experiencing rapid social change, urbanization, increased exposure to mass media. Traditional systems are rapidly changing, initiation ceremonies are less common and, increasingly, children are staying on at school. Adolescence in many developing countries is beginning to resemble the situation in industrialized countries.

Health education and the pre-school child

As I described above, the first five years of a child's life are extremely important for the development of the child. The foundations of physical, intellectual, social, emotional and language development are being laid. Health education can be carried out with the pre-school child in many ways. One important way is through educational programmes reaching the 'caretakers' of the child. These caretakers might include the parents – usually the mother – and other members of the family involved in decision-making on child-care, including the father, grandparents or older brother and sister. Educational programmes can involve:

- family-life education provided in schools, preparing pupils for future roles as parents;
- education on child care and child development provided for parents as part of ante-natal education or at child health clinics;
- non-formal education of parents in the home and community settings such as women's groups, fathers' clubs, churches and other organizations;
- public education directed at families involving various forms of media including books, leaflets, magazine articles, radio and television programmes providing advice on parenthood.

It is possible to reach pre-school children directly through crèches or nurseries. These might be run by government, private and voluntary agencies and provide care and support for children for all or part of the day. Some nurseries are able to care for very young children from the first few months. Others do not take

171

Pre-school provisions improve child health and development by

- enabling mothers to work and increase family income

- releasing young girls from child care duties so that they can attend school

- providing opportunities for reaching children with child health and nutrition services including screening, growth monitoring, immunization, child-feeding programmes

- educational opportunities (e.g. for social, emotional, language and intellectual development) for children from poor and deprived communities and laying the foundations for good performance at school

- specific health education activities which encourage healthy routines such as handwashing, care of teeth, nutrition

- providing opportunities to carry out non-formal education with parents on child health and development

Fig. 9.2 Ways in which pre-school provisions can improve child health and development

children until they are 2–3 years old. Crèches and nurseries can benefit the health and development of the pre-school child in many ways as shown in Figure 9.2.

Many people think that learning must always involve formal 'teaching' sessions. They treat play as a way of keeping a child amused, filling in time and do not consider it very important. However, one of the most important ways in which pre-school children develop is through play. While playing, children learn new things including: exploring movements by using hands and the body and balancing; developing powers of thinking; finding out how to express themselves; using imagination; and learning how to get on with others.

Play is an activity that takes place naturally. For example, even in traditional rural communities, it is common to see young children playing at adult roles with pretend stoves and dolls. Most children have curiosity and interest in the world around them. Without any special effort they will involve the people around them and make use of whatever objects they come into contact with, such as leaves, twigs and household objects.

If play is such a natural process, why then do we need to make a special effort to promote it? Parents and services are often unaware of how their children's development can be helped through play. The most important resource is the willingness of adults to spend time doing things with young children – it is not necessary to spend large amounts of money on expensive toys. It is possible to make simple and very effective 'junk toys' from everyday items such as plastic bottles and cardboard boxes. Verbal play can involve storytelling, riddles and jokes. Pre-school provisions such as crèches can provide an even wider range of experiences than the home and can expand and stretch a child's experiences.

Play is the best way of introducing ideas about health to the pre-school child. It is possible to introduce basic health concepts through puzzles, stories, songs, acting games, a range of other games, and drawing (see Figure 9.3).

Fig. 9.3 Play and health

Case studies of health education programmes with parents and pre-school children

Backyard nurseries in Kingston, Jamaica In the city of Kingston, it is common to find women on their own bringing up their children. A network of small nurseries has arisen to care for the children and allow the mother to work. The local women who set up these 'backyard nurseries' as small businesses had no special training in the care of children and facilities were often inadequate. The Department of Social and Preventive Medicine in the University of the West Indies set out to upgrade these nurseries without destroying their community-based approach. They provided training for the attendants, helped them to improve the facilities including general surroundings, water and sanitation; and arranged for health workers to visit the nurseries regularly. They also included sessions where the mothers were told about what they could do to promote their children's development.

Mobile crèches, Delhi, India Many poor women in India are building-workers in the cities. Because this involves moving from place to place, it is difficult to find child care and so even quite young children are left to play in dangerous surroundings on

173

the building sites. In 1969 a group of voluntary workers set up a mobile crèche in a tent for children under three years old. From this small beginning a network of mobile crèches has been set up, usually located in donated rooms in nearby buildings. The range of activities undertaken by the project has expanded. They have a crèche for the very young, a nursery class for the older children and elementary classes for children between ages of 6 and 12 who had been unable to attend school because of their travelling lifestyle. A doctor visits each crèche regularly. Adult education sessions are held with the parents. Before carrying out immunization programmes, parents' meetings are held and films are shown to explain the importance of health care.

Integrated Child Development Services Scheme (ICDS) in India The ICDS scheme is a large-scale programme initiated by the Government of India with assistance from UNICEF. Its objectives have been to improve the nutritional and health status of children below six years of age and to lay the foundation for proper psychological, physical and social development of the child. These objectives are reached through a package of services made up of feeding programmes, immunization, health check-ups, referral services, health and nutrition education and non-formal pre-school education. A village-based worker is responsible for enrolling every pre-school child and pregnant woman in her village into the programme. One key feature was the setting up of pre-school centres called ***anganwadis*** (courtyards) as focuses of health, education and nutritional activities including growth monitoring. The ***anganwadi*** worker is encouraged to make follow-up visits to the homes. Evaluations of this large-scale programme have shown that, in some parts of the country, there were improvements in health, nutritional status and immunization coverage. Educational opportunity, as measured by attendance and performance at school, also improved. These evaluations pointed to the importance of continued training and supervision of the village workers, the value of community participation and of ensuring close links with other health personnel.

Day-care centres in Senegal Local women in a rural part of Senegal wanted somewhere to leave their children in safety during the planting season when women and young girls were busy in the fields. They were provided facilities on condition that the women themselves organized the service and met any expenses. The rural women planted a kitchen garden to provide food for their childrens' midday meal and took turns looking after the children and cooking the daily meal. Other communities copied the example and, six years later, by 1978, there were 58 such centres catering for 6004 children. The day-care centres were focal points for community life. They became a meeting point for the community, government and voluntary agencies to work to improve the situation of children in the community. Volunteers among the young people in the community receive special training to help in the community.

Fathers' clubs in Lagos, Nigeria The Institute of Child Health of the University of Lagos set up a Fathers' Club at a clinic in a low-income area of Lagos. The aim of the club was to enlist the support of the fathers in improving and maintaining the health of the family, with particular reference to mothers and pre-school children. Between 30 and 50 fathers met monthly in the evenings. The fathers ran the club themselves. At each meeting there was a talk by the clinic staff and time for the fathers to discuss clinic activities, make complaints and suggestions.

Child-to-Child Programme – worldwide The Child-to-Child Programme is a worldwide network of groups seeking to mobilize schools for health education among children and their communities. One early aim of the programme was to use schoolchildren to reach their younger brothers and sisters. Activities to be carried out with younger children included a range of health interventions, including nutrition, oral rehydration, mobilization for immunization and prevention of accidents. Child development was also an important component and the project has produced activity sheets on: playing with babies, playing with young children, toys and games for young children and making a playground (see later in the chapter for more details of the Child-to-Child Programme).

The school-aged child

There are over a thousand million children of school age in the world. In recent years the developing countries have made great strides in increasing the numbers of children enrolled in primary and secondary schools. In developing countries about 80 per cent of children now enrol in primary or elementary school (ages 6–14) and 60 per cent complete at least four years of school. In March 1990 a world conference held in Bangkok called for a target of *Education for All by the Year 2000*. This proposed educational expansion will provide an exciting opportunity to develop school-based health programmes.

Why are schools important for health?

Schools can create an educated population who are then better able to make use of the health education they receive in later life from sources such as newspapers, radio and leaflets. This is particularly important in the education of women. Many studies have shown that an educated woman is more likely to take steps to improve the health and nutrition of herself and her family.

It can be difficult for health educators to reach adults directly. Only some adults may visit the clinics and health centres. Mass media such as radio are only suitable for simple messages. Schools provide a way of eventually reaching the whole of a population at an early age before adult behaviours such as diet and smoking are established.

Schools can also *directly* influence the health of the school child – through preventive health measures such as immunization and dental health as well as screening programmes for early detection of problems in growth and development.

A school health programme has three components: these are *school health services*; a *health-promoting school environment* and a *school health education programme*. These three components are reinforced by external influences such as support from parents, public education and the primary health care services. See Figure 9.4.

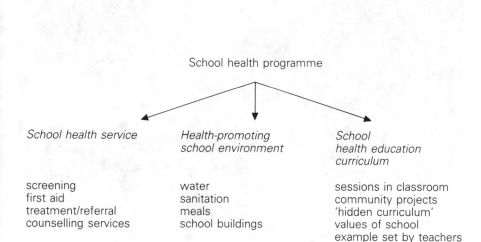

Fig. 9.4 Components of a school health programme

Fig. 9.5 Using schools to improve health

School health services

Depending on local needs and available resources schools can be used for a wide range of important activities that include:

- screening for growth (weight and height), hearing and eyesight;
- immunizations against common childhood diseases, including measles and rubella;
- simple preventive and curative treatment for childhood diseases including roundworms, malaria, schistosomiasis;
- screening for dental health, simple preventive dental services;
- identification of hygiene problems and necessary action, e.g. head-lice infestation;
- counselling for children (and parents) with psycho-social problems affecting their mental health;
- first aid for minor accidents and referral to health services.

Where health workers are scarce, alternatives to doctors and nurses are needed for school health services. Teachers are in close contact with pupils and are in an excellent position to promote health activities. An example of involving teachers in school health programmes is the Khanghaza School Health Programme in Kerala. Teachers in 30 schools were given a short training in first-aid and recognition of common childhood diseases. They were able to treat basic problems, refer children to the health centre and liaise with health services for screening and immunization programmes. Involvement of the teachers in simple first-aid and treatment increased their confidence and credibility to develop health education activities in the school.

The school environment

The environment of the school is important for the health of the schoolchild. It also forms part of the 'hidden curriculum' of the school. If schools do not have good provisions for sanitation, clean water and facilities for hygienic preparation of food, children cannot be expected to take seriously the health education they receive in the classroom.

Clean, safe water is needed both for drinking and the washing of hands. The school environment should be kept clean with bins and pits provided for rubbish. Classrooms must be clean and dry with adequate lighting and ventilation.

School meals can have an important role in the nutrition of the schoolchild and many countries have set up feeding programmes. Food should be prepared in clean conditions by properly supervised cooks.

Sanitation is essential for health. Schools should have latrines that must be clean and properly maintained. In Lesotho in Southern Africa a programme was developed by the Urban Sanitation Improvement Team (USIT) to introduce sanitation into primary schools. USIT gave technical advice to schools on construction of latrines and helped to supervise construction. A 'Ten Point Programme' was developed that listed key points for use of the latrines, reporting of problems and accompanying hygiene measures such as handwashing. These points were also included in a song, wallchart and tape–slide programme for use in the classroom.

The school health education programme

Timetabled lessons and projects in health education

In many countries, only a small proportion of children go on to secondary school. So, to reach everyone, there should be a planned comprehensive curriculum with timetabled sessions in health education, starting from the first year of primary school and extending up to secondary school. These sessions can include classroom activities and practical activities in the community, such as making a survey of local water supplies.

The Child-to-Child Programme encourages children to undertake community projects (see description below). Older children can be selected as 'health guides' and are then involved in teaching younger pupils. This powerful health education technique is called peer-teaching and relies for effectiveness on the fact that younger pupils often have great respect for and try to copy older pupils. Sometimes they listen to the older pupils more than they do their teachers!

Health education as part of other subjects

It is often difficult to find space in the timetable for health education. There may be pressure to emphasize the 'core curriculum' subjects, such as Mathematics, English and Science, that are important for gaining a place in secondary school. A challenging solution to this problem is to build health issues into other subjects. Obvious subjects for including health issues are Home Economics, Biology, Environmental Studies, Physical Education and Agriculture.

However, there are other less obvious subjects that can be used for health education. Local language and English language classes can be used for reading and writing about health. English has a high priority in the 'core' curriculum in many countries. This led the Child-to-Child Programme to develop a set of graded English Language readers containing stories which combine entertainment and health messages on topics ranging from *Good Food, Accidents, Flies, Down with Fever* to *Deadly Habits* (smoking, drinking, drugs and AIDS). Art can be used for painting on health issues, Music for health songs, Drama to show health topics and Religious Education for discussions of values and relationships.

Mathematics provides many opportunities for considering health. A workshop held in Kenya by Child-to-Child has produced a book describing how health examples can be used to teach many basic mathematical concepts including shapes, numbers, graphs, measurement and fractions. Practical activities include counting malaria breeding sites, numbers of children, and of the elderly. The 'Road to Health' growth chart provides a way to introduce graphs and weights and at the same time discuss an extremely important topic in child health. Oral rehydration of children with diarrhoea could form the basis for a science lesson on water and salts.

Out-of-school activities

Many schools have clubs and other out-of-school activities where health topics can be looked at. For example, societies such as the Red Cross, Red Crescent, Boy Scouts and Girl Guides provide opportunities for learning about first aid and other health topics. An advantage is that it is possible to be more relaxed and informal in these out-of-school situations than in the classroom.

The hidden curriculum

The hidden curriculum of the school environment and the teachers' behaviours are an important influence and have already been discussed. What children are taught in the classroom should be practised by the teachers!

Learning methods for school health education

Many people have been critical of traditional teaching approaches in schools that over-emphasize learning facts and passing exams. In health education we usually want to do more than give children facts. We wish to equip them to make decisions, explore attitudes and values and adopt healthy practices both now and in their future lives. Summarized here are the approaches that are increasingly being emphasized in school health education and some examples of school-based health education activities are described on page 181.

Recent approaches in school health education

Child-centred approach – placing the emphasis on meeting the needs of the children, starting with the child's perception of a healthy lifestyle and recognizing that children learn at different rates. The ideas introduced at each level of primary and secondary schooling should reflect the social/emotional, physical and intellectual development of the child.

Active learning methods that encourage exploration and discovery and relate the information presented to everyday life – bridging the gap between home and community.

Problem-solving or 'issue-based' learning which organizes the learning around issues or problems rather than traditional subject disciplines. In this approach, students usually take a health topic and carry out a range of activities in the classroom, at home and in the community. Their finished project might include: songs, drawing, arithmetic, science experiments and story-writing.

Decision-making methods – role plays and exercises where children learn to take decisions. This might include role play where a young person has opportunities to try out different responses to another person's attempt to persuade them to smoke a cigarette, take alcohol or have sex.

Peer teaching methods – which encourage the use of older respected children as 'peer models'. For example, an older child might tell younger children that it is not particularly grown-up to smoke cigarettes.

Self-esteem enhancement – this involves educational approaches that make children develop confidence in themselves and their worth and reduces feelings of failure; children with high self-esteem are more likely to have the confidence to resist pressure from others to engage in risky behaviour.

Teacher-based approaches rather than relying on external visitors – teachers are in the school all the time and know the children better than visitors. Emphasis should be placed on using the teachers themselves as much as possible rather than external visitors to do the health education.

Health education in primary and secondary schools

The most important task in developing a curriculum is to plan the content to match the level and age of the child as she/he progresses through the school. This involves taking into account the various stages of social/emotional, intellectual and physical development that are discussed earlier in the chapter. The primary school is a good place for laying the foundations of health that can be built upon in later schooling. However, in early primary school the child can only grasp simple concepts and ideas. Only later will a child be able to handle more complex and abstract arguments. The spread of content across the different ages may have to be modified for another practical reason. In many countries only a few children go on to secondary school. This means that the health education in the primary school must aim to be as comprehensive as possible to prepare the child for future life.

The secondary school provides an opportunity to build upon the foundations laid by the school health education in the primary school. However, some special problems face health education in secondary schools. Health education may not have been covered well in the primary school, so there may not be a foundation of learning about health to build upon in the secondary school. Emphasis on academic subjects and examinations may restrict time on 'non-essential' subjects like health education. Often health education is carried out in a 'crisis-oriented' approach with visiting speakers brought in to tell pupils of the 'dangers' of alcohol, drugs, tobacco, sex and AIDS. These sessions are not integrated within a broad-based health education programme.

Special problems can be encountered with sex education. Community leaders and parents may not approve of sex education in schools. Teachers can be unwilling to deal with subjects they find embarrassing. There is plenty of evidence of the need for sex education among schoolchildren: a survey of more than 100 Kenyan schoolgirls who became pregnant showed that 65 had never received any information about contraception; studies of how young people learn about sex show that young people often pick up most of their knowledge about fertility and contraception from friends and the media – and much of this is incomplete, misleading and wrong. Myths and misconceptions are common – for example many young people mistakenly believe that pregnancy cannot occur if they are very young, they are having sex for the first time or do not have intercourse very often. Also many are mistaken about when the fertile part of the menstrual cycle occurs. Many countries were reluctant to include sex education in their curriculum but have now changed their position because of the risk of AIDS.

Recent approaches to health education in secondary school children have emphasized a move away from crisis-oriented approaches towards a *planned curriculum* that builds on a foundation laid in primary school. Health education is linked with other developments including counselling, career advisory services and social education. Sex should not be dealt with in isolation. It should be part of a wider *'family life education'* emphasizing responsible relationships, plans for career, preparation for future roles as parents, development of self-esteem and an examination of the pressures from family, friends and society to act in particular ways. With the teenage pupil it is best to use the participatory learning approaches described in Chapter 4. For example, young girls can role-play being asked by a boy to have sex and explore different ways they could respond. Boys can role-play being a girl and becoming pregnant and thus develop understandings of responsible behaviour. A family life education curriculum could consist of the following:

family structures, roles and responsibilities;
growing to maturity, including sexual development;
self-awareness, decision-making and forming relationships;
parenthood, ante-natal care, childbirth, child care;
biology of sexual intercourse, conception and childbirth;
methods of contraception;
population changes in society.

Some examples of school-based health education activities

In **Swaziland** 200 children in 16 primary schools were taught about immunization. Eight radio programmes of 15 minutes' duration were developed to support the classroom activities and one was broadcast each week. Each radio programme started with an immunization song followed by a story by a character called 'Uncle Elijah' who became popular with the children. Children were given workbooks on the six childhood killer diseases.

In **Côte d'Ivoire** teachers and students formed a theatre group and performed sketches on immunization and ORT.

In a low-income area in **India**, poliomyelitis immunization coverage increased from 20 per cent to 90 per cent when school children assumed responsibility for bringing their brothers and sisters to the vaccination post.

In **Zambia** a network of Anti-AIDS clubs were set up throughout the country and these were used to discuss with pupils issues of AIDS, sexually-transmitted diseases and sex education.

In **Ecuador** 34 000 teachers and 150 000 secondary school students provided families with training on child health. A follow-up showed that 50 per cent of families had used ORT and over half said that they had learnt it from a secondary school student.

In **Zimbabwe** a video was produced called *Consequences* exploring through the words of young people the pressures on a schoolgirl that led her to become pregnant and leave school.

In **Jamaica** a support programme was set up for pregnant girls so that they could receive help to look after their child and continue their studies.

The Child-to-Child Programme

The International Year of the Child in 1979 saw the launching of the Child-to-Child Programme which has since expanded to more than 70 countries. According to Hugh Hawes, one of the founders, the Child-to-Child Programme is based on three fundamental assumptions:

1. That primary education becomes more effective if it is linked closely to things that matter most to children and to their families and communities.
2. That education in school and education out of school should be linked as closely as possible so that learning becomes a part of life.
3. That children have the will, the skill and the motivation to help educate each other and can be trusted to do so.

In its early stages, the Child-to-Child Programme placed special emphasis on the idea of using the primary schoolchild to reach out to younger brothers and sisters.

Child-to-Child

Child-to-Child Activity Sheets are a resource for teachers, and health and community workers. They are designed to help children understand how to improve health in other children, their families, and their communities. Topics chosen are important for community health and suit the age, interests and experience of children. The text, ideas and activities may be freely adapted to suit local conditions.

PREVENTING ACCIDENTS

THE IDEA

In some places, as many as two children in a school die each year because of accidents. Many more will be injured. **These accidents need not happen.** Children can help to reduce the number and seriousness of accidents by practising safety at home, out-of-doors and on the road. Children can learn to spot the most common dangers, and understand how these dangers can be avoided or prevented. They should always watch out for the safety of others, particularly smaller children.

Children can also be prepared to help when an accident happens.

Children can talk about the accidents which they have seen happen most often in their community. Different sorts of accidents happen to children who live in different places - in towns, in villages, in rural areas. Identify accidents which have happened in the last six months at home, on the road, anywhere out-of-doors and discuss **why** they happened.

At Home

*   **burns** from cooking pots or lamps, electrical appliances, hot food, boiling water, steam, hot fat (scalds), strong acid or corrosives (like battery acid) which damage the skin;
*   **cuts** from broken glass, rusty pins, rough wood or sharp knives and axes;
*   **obstruction (preventing) of breathing** from swallowing small objects like coins, buttons and nuts;
*   **poisoning** from eating or drinking harmful things;
*   **internal (inside) bleeding** from swallowing sharp objects like razor blades;
*   **electric shock** from touching a broken electrical appliance or electrical wire.

On the Road

*   **death** or injuries like heavy **bleeding, broken bones** and **damage to main organs** of the body (liver, lungs, brain) (*see* Sheet 4.2, **Road Safety**).

In the Playground or Out-of-Doors

*   **burns, cuts and broken bones;**
*   **poisoning** from eating certain plants and berries;
*   **bites** from animals and snakes and stings from bees and other insects;
*   **drowning** in open water or wells.

This sheet can be used together with Sheet No. 4.2, **Road** Safety and Sheet No. 4.3, **First Aid.**

Fig. 9.6 A Child-to-Child worksheet

The approach has now widened to include a wide range of new and exciting approaches for promotion of health in schools.

Table 9.1 Key messages in the Child-to-Child Programme

Personal and community hygiene and safety	Prevent accidents. Care for teeth. Promote neighbourhood hygiene.
Prevention and control of disease	Oral rehydration saves the lives of children with diarrhoea. Learn to recognize danger-signs of illness. Care for sick children.
Child stimulation and development	Play and mental stimulation help children develop. Toys and games can be made that aid growth and development.
Recognizing and helping the handicapped	Children with sight and hearing problems need to be identified and their problems understood.
Prevention of malnutrition	Signs of malnutrition can be recognized and its causes understood. Better feeding is usually possible even though more money may not be available.

Eleven key messages were originally identified and these are shown in Table 9.1. Each message is accompanied by a series of practical activities that would be realistic, interesting and fun for children to undertake. Activity sheets (which are distributed free from the address in Appendix C) were prepared (see Figure 9.6). These encouraged children to:

- understand the main message;
- find out more about the problem in their community through projects and surveys; look for interesting ways to organize and present the information obtained;
- discuss possible solutions with their teacher and fellow pupils;
- apply solutions – including learning any necessary skills, learning how to explain and convince others, taking action in the community;
- evaluate the effect of their actions.

A survey carried out in 1987 of 114 Child-to-Child projects in 39 countries showed that activities undertaken fell into three broad groups. The largest single group of activities were '*outreach projects*' where children applied their knowledge to help others in the community. For example, a report from Kenya described how 'The headmaster, teachers and pupils in our primary school have joined hands to help the children in a handicapped school which is in our community. We have made crutches for the handicapped children who need them. Our children enjoy working with the handicapped children, and the handicapped children enjoy learning with normal children.'

183

Table 9.2 An example of an integrated project approach

Topic: children should be able to establish the relationship between polluted water and disease.

SUBJECT AREAS	ACTIVITIES and TEACHING METHODS
Oral expression	Tell about the sickness.
	Question children about their opinion.
Educational games	Sequence of pictures and/or comic strips about the different phases of diarrhoea: e.g. a child drinks polluted water, has stomach pains, has diarrhoea.
Visits	Go to the health centre, question the nurse.
Mathematical activity	Ask children about diarrhoea among their younger brothers and sisters. Plot the results on a histogram to show how common it is.
Graphics	Ask children to draw pictures of themselves when sick.
Symbolic games	Mime sickness in a simple play.
(drama)	Make puppets and prepare a show.
	Play a scene about the disease and how to treat it with oral rehydration solution.
Songs and stories	Make up a song about water and health.
Reading	Read story from Child-to-Child reader about dirty water.
Science	Discuss nature of water, salts and sugars.
Practical activity	Make up oral rehydration solution for a child with diarrhoea.

The next largest single group were '*enquiry projects*' (28 per cent) where children used Child-to-Child materials and investigations to acquire knowledge that they will use later. One report from Fiji described how: 'As a schoolteacher I and my colleagues have used Child-to-Child materials in health education to advance children's knowledge through reading and through activity. The children were involved in carrying out experiments and in collecting data and other records. Since these activities are child-oriented it gives them a chance for self-discovery.'

The third group consisted of a mixture of approaches where the Child-to-Child materials were used in the classroom and for training of teachers. In another review of Child-to-Child programmes, Audrey Aarons suggested the active learning methods listed here. An example of a project-based activity is given at the top of this page.

Some 'Child-to-Child' methods for school health education

Chalk and talk: using the black-board or 'chalkboard'; making lists, e.g. foods in the market; classifying information; preparing action plans, e.g. for a clean-up programme; writing out instructions; measuring things and summarizing information on a graph or chart.
Picture talks: drawing pictures on chalkboard, on paper; cutting out pictures for flannelgraphs, flip charts, comic books; story rolls; asking questions about each picture; making a mural (large wall painting).

Storytelling: telling stories at class, school assemblies, while waiting at health centres; telling stories to younger children; making pictures to accompany stories; putting pictures in flip charts and flannelgraphs.

Songs: making up songs about health topics.

Dramatizations: acting-out stories; dressing up and performing plays; using role play to imagine what it is like being in a situation; making and performing puppet plays to other children and the community.

Reading and writing: reading health stories; comics, newspapers, magazines, posters and pamphlets; writing health stories and messages; writing letters about local activities; making health posters; making record cards; preparing school newspapers and notice boards.

Experiments and demonstrations: making, doing, growing, weighing, measuring things; observing things, discussing them, telling others about them, portraying them in dramas, plays, puppet shows or exhibitions.

Projects and campaigns: in the school and community.

Setting up a school health programme

A starting-point is for health workers, parents and teachers to meet and discuss their common interests and needs. Health education is usually in the school syllabus but may not be taught well or given much priority. Parents often want their children to do well at school and gain academic qualifications and can resist any move away from traditional academic subjects. However, you can use the argument that a healthy child performs better at school, to persuade education authorities, teachers and parents to support the expansion of health-promoting activities.

From these discussions you can formulate a policy for developing a school health programme covering each of the three areas described above: school health services, school environment and health education. Some of the questions you will have to ask to develop your curriculum are listed below.

Questions to ask when planning a school health programme

- What do parents, teachers, pupils, community leaders and health workers feel about the need to expand health education in schools? What topics do they feel should be a priority? How do they feel about each topic area including sensitive subjects such as sex education?
- Is there already a health education curriculum? How much scope for improvement is there through teacher training and improved resources within the present curriculum? Does the curriculum have to be changed? Can this be done locally or is the curriculum determined at the national level?
- How should the content be organized to ensure an integrated comprehensive curriculum rather than a crisis-oriented approach? How much time should be allocated to timetabled sessions on health education? How much emphasis should be placed on expanding health education within existing subjects such as mathematics, English and science? How can the curriculum be organized in each school year to meet the child's changing physical, social/emotional and intellectual development as well as health needs? Should health education be assessed in examinations? How can the curriculum reflect the needs of the community and the national culture?

- Do existing teaching methods in the schools need to be changed to allow effective school health education? What scope is there for project-based activities, field visits and 'Child-to-Child' activities?
- What preparation do teachers need to undertake school health education? How should this training be organised? What support do they need, such as educational materials, and how can these be provided?
- What scope is there for expanding out-of-school activities such as clubs and sports to support the school health programme?
- What improvements in the school infrastructure of water supply, toilets, waste disposal and school meals are needed to support the educational activities?
- What organizational structure, such as a school health committee, is needed to bring together interested groups such as health workers, parents and teachers, to plan and implement school health-promotion activities?

A good example of a national curriculum development approach is the school health education programme in Uganda. A national committee was set up with representatives from the Ministry of Health, Ministry of Education and other interested groups. It was decided to locate the health education within the existing science curriculum and make it an examinable subject. The curriculum was tested in 20 schools and covers topics such as nutrition, safe-water sanitation, immunization, the treatment of common diseases, the prevention of accidents and AIDS. A series of 'training of trainers' workshops was held to create a network of trainers. These trainers went on to run workshops for teachers in every district on how to implement the new curriculum. With the assistance of UNICEF, a set of attractively-produced support materials were produced, including wall charts and a teachers' guide.

Some people criticize centralized curriculum development approaches because they do not always meet needs of local communities. They also represent a 'top-down' approach and miss out on the opportunities presented when teachers, parents and health workers work together to develop school health programmes. In a district-based approach to curriculum development in the South Indian State of Kerala, one teacher was selected from each of 30 schools. They were responsible for development of the school health programme in their school, for coordinating health education activities and supporting the work of other teachers. The teachers were trained on simple treatment and prevention of local diseases, first aid and a range of health education activities including project-based health education approaches. On return to their schools they set up school health committees, attended sick children, started screening activities and set up a variety of school health education activities in the school and community.

If you cannot work at the national or district level you can still work among the schools in your immediate community. If you have not had much experience of schools it is essential to talk to local teachers and see how they feel about health education and what could be done at the local level. Find out what scope there is for improving the quantity and quality of health promotion activities within the present curriculum. A list of helpful books on school health education and some addresses of resource agencies are given in the Appendixes.

Reaching children out-of-school

Out-of-school children include the following groups each with their distinct needs:

- schoolchildren in their spare time;

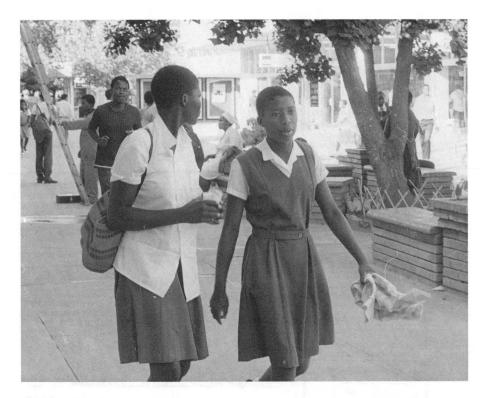

Fig. 9.7 Out-of-school youth

- children who have left school early and are now working, e.g. children of poor landless families in rural areas who are needed for daily activities such as collecting firewood, looking after animals and caring for children;
- children who have never gone to school at all – these could be children orphaned by wars and disease, or deserted by their parents through poverty; also important are the growing numbers of '*street children*' in cities of Latin America, Africa and Asia who earn money from petty trading, parking cars, and in some situations theft and child prostitution.

When they leave school, young people become more independent from their parents and begin to earn money that they may spend going out to bars and discos. They are more likely to be sexually active than schoolchildren at the same age.

Young people out-of-school are one of the most difficult groups to reach. If they attend youth clubs or church groups, educational activities can be carried out in these informal locations. However, many young people do not attend clubs and special approaches are needed to reach these groups.

Young people in urban areas are often interested in music and have their 'youth culture' with distinctive styles of clothing, hair and music. In Uganda a video was made of a song and drama on AIDS produced by a musician who was looked up to and regarded highly by young people. This approach was also used in the pop record made by 'Tatiana and Johnny' described in Chapter 7 on popular media. In Swaziland the National AIDS Committee carried out a survey

Fig. 9.8 A page from *Action* comic in Zimbabwe

of young people to find out which radio programmes they listened to, and used this information to help decide how best to plan their educational strategy.

One advantage of educational programmes outside school is that it is possible to be much more informal and relaxed than in school or in the presence of parents. It is a good opportunity to use the participatory learning methods described in Chapter 4 including group discussion, games and role-plays. Young people will want to show independence from their parents and will expect to be taken seriously. Indeed, if they have been able to survive in the difficult environment of a city street, they will know a great deal already about life and resent being talked to like children. Their experiences are a resource to build upon. If their participation is encouraged, they will be able to suggest appropriate methods and strategies for reaching other young people. Some promising approaches for working with young people are to:

- use people that young people look up to, such as singers or football players to speak on health issues;
- ask popular music groups to perform songs about health issues;
- use young people as fieldworkers that youths will listen and respond to;
- involve young people themselves in producing a drama about their lives and situation;
- train a group of young volunteers to carry out informal health education in the bars and discos where the young people go;
- produce magazines and comics on health topics;
- include health issues in the initiation ceremonies that are carried out for both boys and girls in many countries and serve as traditional forms of sex education.

Summary – promoting the health of children and young people

There is enormous scope for expanding and improving health education activities for pre-school children, schoolchildren and out-of-school youth and if you wish to take this further you can consult the list of reading and addresses provided in the Appendixes. It is possible to draw the following general conclusions.

1. There is a need to expand the quantity and quality of educational interventions directed at young children. Special efforts are needed to meet the needs of those groups in society with the worst health: usually the poorest; children of parents with few educational qualifications; children who have missed out on school; and girls.
2. Health education should bridge the gap between school and community through relevant content, community projects and involvement of parents and community leaders; the curriculum should consider health problems in the community and the influence of the family, friends and community.
3. Educational methods should match the developmental stage of the child; they should go beyond just giving facts and be action-oriented and enquiry-based; and develop thinking ability and decision-making. Teachers will need training and support to enable them to introduce these methods.
4. School-based programmes should be supported by other interventions to reach those children not attending school.
5. Educational programmes directed at children should be part of a comprehensive community-based primary health care approach with the full participation of health workers, teachers, parents, pupils and the community.

Fig. 9.9 The Karate Kid in Mexico

Some examples of working with out-of-school youth

CORA, Mexico A youth programme called CORA gave lectures on sex education to parents. It also sponsored annual theatre competitions open to young people aged 12–22. The contestants write, produce and act in their own plays. Local officials and celebrities judge the performances and prizes are awarded. The plays have dealt with all areas of concern to young people, from sexual development to political corruption. In the five years between 1980 and 1985 over 6100 youths performed to more than 270 000 people. Even hard-to-reach youths such as street children have participated.

Karate Kid – South America The emergence of AIDS has raised many people's concerns about street children – especially because a growing number of them are forced into making a living through child prostitution. An interesting programme in Mexico was sponsored by the organization Street Kids International. They produced a cartoon film on video that featured a hero character, *Karate Kid* and used it with street children in educational projects on AIDS.

BRAC – Bangladesh In Bangladesh a voluntary agency, BRAC, started a non-formal primary education programme for children who have dropped out of schools. They offer two courses. The first course, lasting three years, is for children aged 8–10 and places special emphasis on reaching girl drop-outs. The second course, lasting two years, is for 11–14 year-olds. The goal is to develop functional literacy, with emphasis on numeracy and social studies. The social studies course consists of health, nutrition, hygiene, sanitation, safety and first-aid. By mid-1990 there were 67 000 students enrolled in over 2000 schools.

Copperbelt Health Education Project The Copperbelt Health Education Project in Zambia developed an educational programme among street children. They ran a one-week workshop for street children, that included the following sessions: staying healthy (covering AIDS, STDs, drug abuse, alcohol abuse and cigarette-smoking and a visit to the local hospital); staying within the law (including a visit to the local police station); going back to the land (a visit to a farm training centre); running a successful

190

small business (including basic arithmetic and accountancy); and locally available skills training opportunities.

LINGAP Centre, Philippines The LINGAP centre in Manila in the Philippines gives alternative education for street children and abused children. Children work in groups of 10–12 with games, role playing and group sharing. They learn to help each other and use materials from the Child-to-Child Programme which they take to others outside the centre.

Grapevine project, London Young people are strongly influenced by their friends and this can be made use of in your health education. The approach of training young volunteers was used successfully in the 'Grapevine' family-planning health education project among young people. The young people carried out informal health education on a range of topics with their peers in pubs, discotheques and concerts. A similar programme of youth volunteers in Hong Kong – called the 'Society of New Generations' (SONG) provide family life education to groups of young people in workplace and community settings.

---

10. Politics and health

In looking at health problems and their causes we have seen that there are limits to what can be achieved by working at the individual level. In particular, I have emphasized the danger of *victim-blaming* – where we focus our educational activities on the individual and ignore external factors such as pressure from others, poverty, lack of facilities and opportunities for change. It is not enough to help people make decisions. We have to make it easier for them to make healthy choices.

In the list below are a few of the political, social and economic factors that can influence health and make healthy choices. These include government policies concerning:

military expenditure and war;
human rights;
actions that increase poverty, social inequalities and unemployment;
policies affecting the status of women and children;
policies leading to harmful environmental changes, e.g. deforestation, pesticides, dumping of toxic wastes;
policies affecting urbanization, availability of adequate housing, water and sanitation;
costs of foods, subsidies for agriculture, imports;
pricing and availability of basic commodities such as foods, clothing, soap, transport;
legislation to remove hazards from the workplace;
pricing of harmful substances such as tobacco, alcohol and baby milk substitutes;
advertising of health-damaging products;
actions by multinational companies;
spending on health care and education;
accessibility and appropriateness of health care services and commitment to primary health care.

Most of these take us outside the traditional work of health services. As individuals, we often feel helpless when faced with the immense task of trying to influence our own government or other countries. Yet these factors are crucial to the creation of a healthy society. If we take seriously our task of promoting health we cannot simply walk away from these responsibilities and say that they are not our concern.

It was in response to these concerns that many people became dissatisfied with the traditional view of health education that put too much emphasis on the individual and not enough on community and government action. In Chapter 1, I described the broader concept of *health promotion* that includes health education as well as actions to influence government policies that concern health.

Some of the different ways in which communities can come together to work for change were described in Chapter 6. In particular, I discussed how the ideas of Paulo Freire could be applied to develop the critical awareness of disadvantaged

192

groups and their ability to challenge and change their surroundings. The use of drama for raising consciousness and stimulating social action was described in Chapter 7. This chapter will look at examples of individuals and groups influencing governments and working at the national and international level for political and social action.

Nutrition and food policy

In the past, nutrition education has tended to emphasize the individual person and his or her choice of food. However, as shown in Figure 10.1, the individual is really at the end-point of a series of stages from cultivation, marketing, purchasing, food processing and sharing-out in the home. The actual food received by a member of a family is the result of many different factors, only some of which are under a person's control. Some factors such as food availability, income and women's time are seasonal and change during the year.

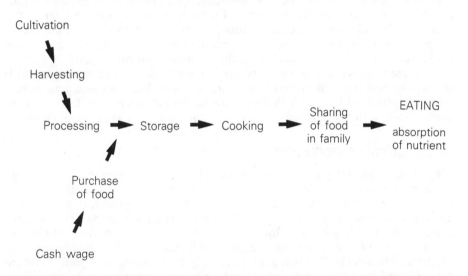

Fig. 10.1 The food pathway

Nutrition and food consumption are influenced by national policies. Most important of these are the prices paid to farmers and whether incentives are given to plant particular crops. For example, cash crops may be encouraged rather than food crops. In the colonial period many countries such as Ghana, Kenya and Mauritius were encouraged to devote their best land to cash crops for the colonial power and this pattern continued after independence. Attempts to transfer more land to cultivation of food have been made difficult by the need to obtain foreign exchange to pay back debts to the West and the fall in prices of cash crops. Furthermore, cash crops can themselves be health-damaging, as you will see when the issues of smoking and tobacco control are discussed later in the chapter.

Governments often try to keep prices of foods down so that the poor can afford them. In 1987, food riots took place in Zambia when prices of maize in the towns were increased beyond the reach of the urban poor. But keeping prices down can have wider effects. Paying farmers more can lead to greater earning power in rural areas and improvement in facilities and services that might encourage people to stay in the rural areas rather than migrate to the cities. Of course, increased prices for rural farm produce must be accompanied by measures such as improved wages for landless labourers and land reforms if the benefits are going to reach the rural poor.

Measures which increase agricultural productivity can have harmful effects on health. The overuse of pesticides is affecting the ecological balance, leading to increased resistance to insecticides of the malaria mosquito and poisoning of agricultural workers (WHO estimate that there are approximately 500 000 cases of pesticide poisoning including 5000 deaths every year). Large-scale irrigation projects have had some unexpected side-effects. These include providing breeding-sites for malaria mosquitos and the snails that spread schistosomiasis.

The importing, marketing and advertising of foods can have implications for health. In West Africa, locally-produced palm oil is rich in vitamin A and, unlike imported cooking oil, does prevent blindness from vitamin A deficiency. Importing of cooking oil has led to reduced production of palm oil. Consumer products, e.g. drinking chocolate, are heavily advertised and promoted as modern. Many processed foods are not directly harmful (although, as you will see later in this chapter, baby-milk substitutes are definitely harmful). However, they encourage people to spend money on expensive prestige products when the same money could buy a substantial amount of locally-produced, nutritious food.

Agriculturalists and economists dealing with pricing and import controls rarely take health and nutrition issues into account. Yet their decisions have a profound effect on health. A challenge for health educators is to learn to work more closely with these groups to develop food policies that promote health.

Intersectoral collaboration

Many health issues require the involvement of different government departments or 'sectors'. Government departments and non-governmental organizations dealing with housing, social welfare, education, agriculture, employment, industry, rural development, communications, women's affairs, youth and transport can all affect health in their different ways. Intersectoral collaboration is an essential element of the concept of primary health care and health promotion described in the early chapters of this book. You will almost certainly find yourself in a position where you will need to involve other departments in your programmes or influence their policies so that they support your health promotion activities.

There are examples of successful intersectoral collaboration that we can learn from. In the South American country of Colombia on 23 June, 28 July and 25 August 1984 one million children were vaccinated against diphtheria, whooping cough, tetanus, polio and measles. A coordination committee was set up for this 'National Vaccination Crusade'. The participating organizations included: the Ministry of Health; the Ministry of the Interior who involved the governors and mayors of the 950 municipalities; the Ministry of Education who mobilized 200 000 teachers to support the programme; the Ministry of Communication who mobilized televisions for spots and for telephone communication; the Ministry of Defence who provided air, sea and river transportation; the Institute of Social Security, the Catholic Church, the Red Cross, the Boy Scouts, cultural groups and private enterprise.

The Colombian programme provides an example of the *Social Mobilization* approach on a national scale. It was able to involve a wide range of organizations because of the support from the national leadership and the involvement of the President of the Republic. A visit from the Director of UNICEF, James Grant, also helped to unite the different organizations. Most important, there was a simple clear aim that everyone could accept to be important and worthwhile.

Although there is widespread agreement about the need for intersectoral collaboration, it can be very difficult to get everyone to work together. Each agency may have different priorities. Staff may have a narrow view of health as something concerning only hospitals and medicines and may not recognize the role their institution can play. They may be suspicious that you are trying to take some of their budget and 'invade' their 'territory'. The priority of many bureaucracies and administrators is often to protect their own organization!

Campaigns, such as the one described above in Colombia, are one way of uniting different groups for a short intensive action to meet agreed objectives. Sustained collaboration between agencies needs a political commitment from the senior management at district and national levels. Some useful strategies to create mutual understanding, enthusiasm and commitment to work together are listed below.

- When you are trying to involve someone from another department don't just think what you want that person to do for you. See if you can think of ways in which involvement in your programme might benefit *their* work. Find out what are the special needs, pressures and tasks facing that person and what outcomes of joint action might be perceived as beneficial to them. Are there pressures from their senior management that you need to know about? Much can be achieved informally at a local level, though: mutually helping each other; supporting each other's activities; and sharing equipment, skills and transport.
- Hold orientation meetings for persons from different departments at the beginning of your health education programme and provide opportunities for participation, discussion and sharing of thoughts on future activities.

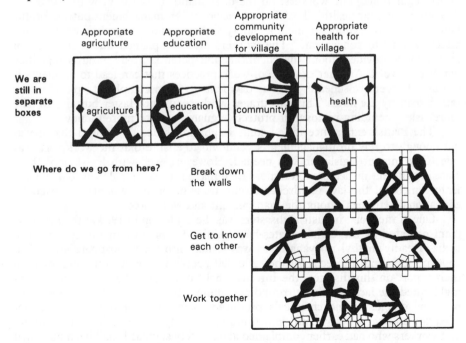

Fig. 10.2 Inter-sectoral collaboration – breaking the barriers

195

- In any initial training, continuing education or workshop activities you are involved in, encourage a *multidisciplinary* mix of participants. Use participatory training methods that encourage exploring of different perspectives, agreements on respective roles, building of mutual trust and a strategy for joint action.
- Create regular opportunities where the different fieldworkers can meet in an informal setting and exchange information on current activities and problems.

Health and safety at work

Work can be dangerous for your health. Depending on their jobs, workers might be exposed to a variety of hazards that include chemicals, dust, vibration, noise and dangerous machinery. We have only just begun to realize the harmful effects of many of these. Learning has been a painful process at the expense of many unnecessary deaths.

In 1974 Britain passed its Health and Safety at Work Act that made it law for companies to take action to ensure that their workplace did not have any hazards. Companies had to have a written health and safety at work policy that outlined their strategy and had to appoint a health and safety officer. They were also encouraged to recognize safety representatives nominated by the trade unions and allow them to be released for training. Government officials, called factory inspectors, were given power to enforce this legislation.

This law led to many educational activities. The UK Trade Union Council set up courses for safety representatives that included the understanding of hazards at the workplace and the nature of the new laws. From the beginning, two opposite perspectives emerged. The management often would blame accidents on 'careless' workers who failed to pay attention, did not wear protective clothing such as eye goggles or ear muffs, took short-cuts in work procedures and broke safety regulations. The workers, on the other hand, took the view that 'work is dangerous for your health'. They blamed accidents on management putting profits before safety by failing to include safety features and using shift-work which affects ability to concentrate. The workers also complained about the lack of information provided about the chemicals and potential toxic hazards that they handled at work. Another example of work practices that can lead to accidents is the use of incentive schemes such as payment per item completed ('piece' work) rather than by the hour. This encourages workers to work faster but also to take more risks, including removal of protective guards to earn more money.

The British experience raised some important issues. It showed that it was not enough to rely on management's good-will to ensure that the workplace was safe. Government legislation was needed. However, even with legislation, there were insufficient inspectors to do more than make the occasional visit to a factory. Enforcement of the law required a strong trade-union movement supported by educational activities among the management and workforce.

One of the worst industrial disasters was the explosion in 1984 at the pesticide plant operated by the United States-based Union Carbide Company at Bhopal in India. Deadly methyl isocyanate gas was leaked into the atmosphere and killed 2500 persons and injured a further 200 000 people in the surrounding area. In their report on this disaster, the International Conference of Free Trade Unions highlighted the fact that the surrounding community was kept ignorant about the potential danger of the chemicals produced. Safety precautions were also not adequate and there was insufficient training in safety. Most serious, they found that workers who had earlier complained about safety standards had been punished by transfer to lower-paying jobs.

196

The International Conference of Free Trade Unions made recommendations which, if implemented, could prevent such disasters in future. These included:

- Workers, trade unions and the general public must be given the full facts about the hazards of any chemical plant, the steps taken to prevent accidents and what must be done if an accident does happen.
- The basic rights of workers and their trade unions should be respected within chemical plants. Workers should be able to select their safety representatives through their trade unions. And the workers must have the right, without any fear of reprisal, to refuse any task that they believe might endanger themselves or the public.

One criticism of educational activities at the workplace is that they tend to concentrate on occupational health. Many health educators have argued that a broader view of health at the workplace is needed. This should include issues such as stress, alcohol consumption, canteen food, smoking policy, crèches for children, and counselling policy. The workplace provides a good opportunity for reaching out to people on a range of issues affecting their lives. Recent workplace health education activities in the United Kingdom have included setting up alcohol policies, changing canteen menus, screening pregnant women at work and setting up policies to cover HIV and AIDS.

The issue of health and safety at work in developing countries is only just receiving attention. A particularly difficult problem is the weak state of many trade unions that makes it easy for management to say that they cannot afford safety measures. Governments are often unwilling to enforce safety regulations on foreign-owned factories who might move to another country with fewer restrictions. As long as there is poverty and the threat of unemployment, people will be willing to work long hours in poor facilities, cramped conditions, with dangerous equipment and exposed to hazardous chemicals.

Tobacco and smoking

The production and sale of cigarettes are controlled by a small group of multinational companies. Now that health education programmes in industrialized countries have been successful in reducing smoking, these companies are trying to expand sales of cigarettes in developing countries. They are encouraged by the low levels of health education on smoking, lack of controls on advertising, the increasing incomes of people in the cities and eagerness of governments to have income from tax on tobacco sales. The brands of cigarettes often have much higher levels – often double – of tar and nicotine than the same brands of cigarettes in industrialized nations where cigarettes with such high levels are banned.

In the figure 10.4, I have detailed some of the preventive measures that have been adopted to control smoking and the barriers faced.

The tobacco companies and their allies are very powerful and influential. Even in industrialized countries it has been difficult to act. In 1985 over US$ 2000 million were spent by the tobacco industry promoting their products; the amount spent by government on health education on tobacco is less than the tobacco industry spends *in a single day*.

Tobacco companies claim that their cigarette advertising is not aimed at encouraging people to smoke, only to switch to their particular brand. However, a careful look at cigarette advertisements shows that this is untrue. Often the advertisements associate cigarettes with modern life, sports, outdoor activities and having fun. In Europe, where advertising of cigarettes has been banned by the

Fig. 10.3 Tobacco advertising in Nigeria

increasing taxes
advertising controls
banning sponsorship
age limits on purchase
warning on packets

public education
school health education

stop smoking clinics
self-help groups

alternative crops
   for tobacco farmers
alternative jobs for
   tobacco workers

pressure groups
direct action

preventing people from
starting to smoke

encouraging smokers
to stop

ensuring those who
stop don't give up

gain support for
anti-smoking laws

OPPOSING INTERESTS
tobacco industry
farmer's lobby
shareholders
finance ministries

Fig. 10.4 Tackling the smoking epidemic

government, tobacco companies have switched to sponsorship of events, especially sports. The name of the event has the name of the cigarette brand which is also displayed prominently on billboards. So every time pictures are shown, or the name of the competition is announced, publicity is given to the tobacco company.

Health educators have been active on smoking for a long time but with only a small part of the money that is available to the tobacco industry. Initial health education concentrated on giving medical facts, but increasingly attractively-produced and pre-tested advertisements are being produced that also directly criticize the cigarette companies.

The UK-based Action on Smoking and Health ('ASH') provides an example of the work of a *pressure group* involved in public education and influencing media coverage and policymakers. Others have despaired of the reluctance of governments to act on controlling and have taken *direct action* that is outside the law. For example, in Australia a group of health educators started writing slogans on the billboards containing the health education advertisements. They called themselves Billboard Utilizing Graffitists Against Unhealthy Promotion, or *BUGA UP*. The name itself was a joke as 'bugger up' is a colloquial term for ruining or spoiling. The slogans were funny and used humour to challenge the images of health, fitness and sophistication on the advertisements. The public found their slogans funny, and newspapers and television gave them publicity and support. The tobacco companies were reluctant to take the members of the group to law court. Newspaper and television reporting of the proceedings of a trial would only provide further publicity about health hazards of smoking.

Governments can be reluctant to pass laws banning tobacco because it will affect their income. For example, almost half the collected tax in Malaysia comes from cigarette sales and in Brazil $100 million per month are collected in cigarette taxes. In Malawi at least half of the export earnings come from the export of tobacco. Many vested interests have to be overcome to deal with the smoking epidemic!

The promotion of bottlefeeding by the infant food industry

In the late 1960s a disturbing trend in many developing countries was observed. Many mothers were turning to bottlefeeding with disastrous consequences for the health of their babies. Lack of water and of hygienic facilities for sterilizing bottles and teats, as well as over-dilution of the baby milk powders led to babies dying from diarrhoea and malnutrition. *A bottlefed baby in a developing country is fourteen times more likely to die in its first year of life than a breastfed one.*

This trend to bottlefeeding was taking place for several reasons. Working mothers found it difficult to combine breastfeeding with a full-time job. Hospitals and maternity wards often found bottlefeeding more convenient to their routines. A widespread belief was that poor mothers had insufficient milk (although, in reality, fewer than one in a hundred mothers has a medical problem that prevents them from breastfeeding their babies). Many also believed that bottlefeeding was modern and better for their babies. These beliefs had arisen for several reasons. In films and magazines bottlefeeding often appeared and breasts were shown as objects of sex. Mothers wishing to breastfeed were discouraged by maternity hospital procedures such as the separation of the mother from her baby, free samples of baby milk and lack of support by trained staff for women experiencing feeding difficulties.

But the most important reasons for the rise in bottlefeeding came from the promotional activities of multinational baby food companies such as Nestlé, Glaxo and Meiji. Their radio, television and billboard advertisements, as well as brightly-decorated cans of milk, promoted the image of bottlefeeding as safe and modern, and undermined women's confidence in breastfeeding. Baby milk companies carried out other promotional activities, including giving free samples of baby milk and advertising in hospitals. Some companies even used sales promotion persons dressed in white coats like health workers.

In the 1970s health workers throughout the developing world began to express concern at the way the infant food manufacturers were promoting bottlefeeding. Charities, consumer groups and development agencies including UNICEF and WHO took up the case. Health workers and women's groups such as the National Childbirth Trust in the United Kingdom were beginning to campaign for a return to breastfeeding in developed countries, so there was the formation of a link and common understanding between countries. An extended international campaign was set up to try to control the activities of the infant food manufacturers. Actions taken included lobbying politicians, boycotts and law-suits (see the timetable on pages 202–3).

An important result of the campaigning was the *International Code for the Marketing of Breast Milk Substitutes* whose provisions included:

- *no free samples or supplies* to be given to mothers or maternity hospitals;
- *no promotion in hospitals* – company posters and literature advertising infant milk products are not allowed in health care facilities;
- *no unscientific promotion to health workers* (including personal gifts) – product literature should be scientific and factual, not promotional;
- *no direct consumer promotion* of infant milk through the mass media and direct contact with customers is prohibited;
- *non-promotional labels* – labels should be non-promotional and include a clear statement on the superiority of breastfeeding and warnings about the hazards of bottlefeeding;
- *scope* – the Code covers breastmilk substitutes, feeding bottles and teats and other products that interfere with breastfeeding.

Individual health workers, development agencies, churches and governments throughout the developing world have mobilized to monitor the implementation of the code. Local self-help groups such as the Baby Milk Action Coalition in the United Kingdom, the Breast Feeding Information group in Kenya and the BUNSO group in the Philippines, have formed. They monitor the activities of infant-food manufacturers, promote breastfeeding among the public, train health workers in breastfeeding counselling and campaign to change maternity hospital practices to encourage breastfeeding. The La Lèche League is a network of women who have groups throughout the world promoting breastfeeding. The International Baby Foods Action Network (IBFAN) acts as an international resource agency (see Appendix C).

The BUNSO group in the Philippines is a good example of a local organization that is facing up to the baby foods industry (the initials BUNSO are an abbreviation for Partnership and Coalition to Save the Infant, in the local language). It is a national coalition of concerned mothers, health workers, consumers, trade union members in the food and drug industry and church groups. They are engaged in the promotion and protection of breastfeeding and in the defence of women and children's rights to proper health and nutrition. BUNSO acts as a 'watchdog' to the milk industry's marketing practices and monitors practices of hospitals, doctors and health workers.

BUNSO was formed in 1981 when Mead Johnson (Bristol Myers) was exposed in the media as dumping out-of-date and vitamin-deficient milk-base in the Philippines. BUNSO led the protest actions and then grew in size until today it acts as an umbrella organization for 65 local action groups representing women, the urban poor, the National Council of Churches and others. BUNSO's activities include: development of community services such as a maternal and child health clinic and a nutrition clinic; community organizing; training; research and documentation; milk code and health advocacy, including public forums and campaigning against advertising of milk and baby foods; support systems including provision of mother's support groups, nurseries in the workplace; hot-line counselling to help mothers to breastfeed. BUNSO was one of the breastfeeding action groups that, as part of IBFAN, participated in the drafting of the Infant Formula Marketing Code.

The vigilance of groups such as BUNSO has helped to expose violations of the Code. For example, a survey by IBFAN in 1988 showed that 13 hospitals surveyed in Thailand received free samples of infant formula, as did 20 out of 23 hospitals in Pakistan and hospitals in Kenya, Singapore and Nigeria. Many of these violations involved multinational companies such as Cow and Gate, Nestlé, Wyeth and Meiji. That same survey found further violations with infant food companies displaying advertisements in hospitals in Pakistan, Sri Lanka, Thailand and Singapore and widespread advertising of baby milks.

The IBFAN survey found 18 baby food manufacturers' labels in Asia that violated the Code either by showing pictures of babies or containing inadequate instructions on making up the baby milk. Despite recommendations of the Pakistan Paediatrics Association, many infant-food companies were giving free antenatal cards, discharge cards and patients folders that contained the name of their

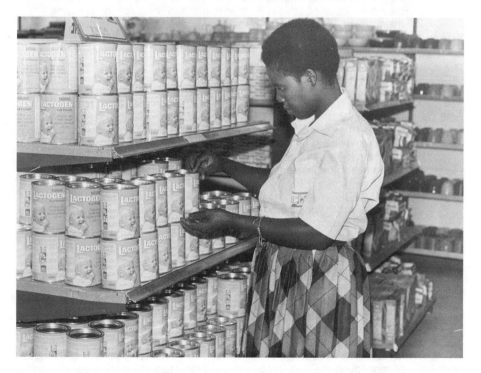

Fig. 10.5 Baby milk advertisements

products. In that same year, 1988, in Thailand the companies Nutricia, AHP, Bristol Myers, Meiji, Abbot and Nestlé all contributed to the costs of New Year's parties at Bangkok Hotels. Later in January doctors in Islamabad and Rawalpindi in Pakistan were treated by the company Meiji to a dinner and music show at the most expensive hotel in town!

The Code should be seen as only a starting-point in the control of this dangerous practice. Action by local groups is needed to make sure the Code is followed.

Action on Baby foods – timetable of main events

1968	Dr Derrick Jelliffe of the Caribbean Food and Nutrition Institute in Jamaica introduces the term 'commerciogenic malnutrition' to describe the impact of industry marketing practices on infant health.
1970	United Nations Protein Calorie Advisory Group (PAG) convenes a meeting on infant feeding that raises concern about industry practices.
1972	International Organization of Consumer Unions (IOCU) submits a draft code of practice for the advertising of infant foods.
1974	UK charity War on Want publishes *The Baby Killer*. In May the Berne Third World Action Group translates the report in Switzerland with German title meaning 'Nestlé Kills Babies' and in July is sued by Nestlé.
1975	Eight baby food companies, including Nestlé, Cow & Gate and Wyeth, form the Industrial Council of Infant Food Industries (ICIFI) and launch their own 'code of ethics'. Further books and films appear exposing malnutrition caused by bottle food.
1976	UN PAG says ICIFI code measures 'do not go far enough'. Final hearing of the Nestlé lawsuit. The Catholic order Sisters of the Precious Blood sue the Bristol Myers Corporation to expose the harmful effects of its promotion of infant foods in the Third World.
1977	US action group INFACT (now called ACTION) launches Nestlé boycott in USA when Nestlé refuses to stop its dangerous marketing practices.
1978	Nestlé boycott spreads to Canada, New Zealand and Australia. Bristol Myers settles out of court and agrees to halt direct consumer advertising of baby milks and end the use of mothercraft nurses. US Senate subcommittee hears testimonies on infant formula problem from Third World health professionals and church representatives. Millions see CBS television film *Into the Mouths of Babes*.
1979	WHO/UNICEF jointly sponsor a meeting in Geneva with over 150 delegates from the UN, governments and NGOs that calls for restriction on infant-food marketing and the infant-food industry representatives agree to accept restrictions. NGOs form the International Baby Food Action Network (IBFAN) to coordinate pressure on the baby-food industry.
1980	Nestlé and three major US baby food companies retract their pledge to abide by the WHO/UNICEF conference recommendations. UK Breast Milk Action Committee (BMAC) launch Nestlé boycott in the UK. WHO and UNICEF prepare a draft code in consultation with government, health workers, consumer groups and the infant-food industry.
1981–82	Nestlé boycott gathers momentum with USA, UK and six other industrialized countries. The International Nestlé Boycott Committee holds regional meetings in Third World to train local groups in techniques of monitoring the baby-food industry, promoting the marketing code and public education on breastfeeding.

1984	Nestlé agrees to implement WHO Code everywhere but in Western Europe.
	Following monitoring of Nestlé, the boycott is suspended.
1985	WHO/UNICEF sponsor a further meeting to amend code to call for prohibition of practice of issuing free samples of baby milk to mothers in maternity wards.
1987–88	IBFAN groups around the world find industry refuses to implement the WHO/UNICEF international code and in some cases are breaking national laws.
1989	On World Consumer Rights day, consumer groups launch boycott of Nescafe in UK, Ireland, Norway and Sweden.

The promotion of non-essential drugs by multi-national companies

A large proportion of national health budgets goes on purchase of drugs. There is increasing concern about the use of drugs that are harmful, unnecessary or which could be available cheaper if bought as 'generic' drugs rather than branded products offered by the multi-national pharmaceutical companies.

In 1988 the World Health Organization calculated that, of the 5 billion people in the world, between 1.3 and 2.5 billion have little or no regular access to essential drugs. At the same time they estimated that 70 per cent of the drugs on the global market are inessential and/or undesirable. The World Health Organization has launched an Essential Drugs Programme. This helps countries to reduce the cost of importing drugs by concentrating on the supply and use of some 250 drugs considered the most essential.

However, the Essential Drugs Programme has been opposed by the pharmaceutical companies, who invest large sums of money in promotion of their drugs through free samples, gifts and incentives to health workers.

One group of drugs that is unnecessary are 'anti-diarrhoeal' medicines. These operate by reducing mobility of the gut. They may relieve symptoms but do not deal with the root causes of diarrhoea. They also distract attention from the life-saving intervention of oral rehydration. Given to young children they can be extremely dangerous. In Pakistan, for example, the company Janson supplied Immodium in droplet form despite the unsuitability of the drug for infants. Despite protests from doctors about the deaths in babies this was causing, the company only finally stopped the availability of the drug after a British television programme exposed the problem in June 1990.

Health Action International is an informal network of some 100 consumer, health, development action and other public interest groups involved in health and pharmaceutical issues in 60 countries around the world. It believes that all drugs marketed should meet real medical needs, have therapeutic advantages, be acceptably safe and offer value for money.

Besides tobacco, baby milks and diarrhoeal medicines, there are other commercial products which can be dangerous to health, including drugs with harmful side-effects, faulty electrical equipment, clothes made from inflammable materials, cosmetics containing harmful chemicals such as skin-lightening creams and eye colouring. The International Organization of Consumers' Unions provides a coordinating function for groups throughout the world who are campaigning for safe products (see Appendix C).

Getting issues on the agenda

A priority in health promotion is to get issues on the 'agenda' of politicians so that they will take them seriously and initiate action. The approach to planning we often see in textbooks is one where priorities are decided according to needs. For example, we might look at prevalence of the disease, trends, seriousness and effect on mortality and morbidity. We might also consider the cost of treatment, feasibility of prevention and felt needs of the community. However, decisions by politicians and government officials are rarely made according to this 'rational' planning model. They are usually made in response to different pressures according to the *status quo* – what has been the practice up to now; influence of friends; allocation of funds from the central government; influence of pressure groups such as professional bodies, commercial companies; trade unions and political parties; external pressures such as prices of imported goods, wishes of aid donor organisations such as the World Bank and the International Monetary Fund; newspapers and television; and public opinion.

Priorities are usually based on short-term pressures and rarely consider longer-term issues such as health and environment. Of course we cannot expect health to be the only issue that governments have to consider. But we can try to influence the public to support health promotion and ensure that politicians are fully informed about the health implications of their decisions.

Forms of protest and action

Those campaigns described above used many different approaches to influence politicians and multinational companies. I have listed on page 205 many different forms of direct action, protest and campaigning approaches (this list is adapted from a longer list of methods of non-violent action prepared by the American Peace activist Gene Sharp). They have been used in campaigns on a wide range of issues including health. Which ones do you think you could apply to bringing attention to a health issue in your community?

The impact of the different methods listed on page 205 depends a great deal on the nature of the health issue and the extent to which the action captures the imagination of the politicians, the media and the public. You can refer to Chapter 8, which describes the type of activities or 'media events' that catch the interest of newspapers, radio and television and explains how to write a press release. People's imagination will be drawn by striking and symbolic acts and the honesty, conviction and sacrifice of those taking action.

One person famous for use of non-violent protests was the Indian *Mahatma Gandhi*. The methods he used to fight injustice and advance the cause of freedom for India are well worth studying as models of action. He called his approach *satyagraha* which means 'truth force'. He used a range of methods including hunger strikes, boycotts, sit-ins, strikes, mass 'stay at homes' and *civil disobedience* – which is the deliberate breaking of laws and being willing to go to prison for causes that one's conscience feels to be just.

Forms of protest and persuasion

Formal statements
public speeches
letter of opposition/
of support
declaration from an
organization
signed public
statement
declaration of
intention
group or mass
petition

**Communication
with a wider
audience**
slogans, symbols
banners, posters
and displays
leaflets, pamphlets
and books
newspapers and
journals
records, television
and radio

**Group
representation**
sending a
deputation
presenting a mock
award
group lobbying
picketing

**Symbolic public
acts**
display or wearing of
symbols
prayer and worship
delivering symbolic
objects
destruction of one's
own property
symbolic lights,
e.g. candles
display of portraits

**Pressure on
individuals**
frequent visits
letter-writing
personal approaches
vigils

Drama and music
humorous sketches,
jokes
performance of
plays and music
singing

Processions
marches and
parades
religious
processions
pilgrimages
honouring the dead
mock funerals
demonstrating at
funerals
homage at burial
places

Public assemblies
assemblies of
protest and support
protest meetings
teach-ins

**Withdrawal and
renouncing**
walkouts
silence
renouncing honours
turning one's back

Boycotts
boycotting of
meetings
withdrawing
membership from
institutions
stay at home
total personal non-
cooperation
consumer boycott

Strikes
protest strike
industry strike
selective strike
general strike

Civil disobedience
slow compliance
sitdown
civil disobedience

**Other non-violent
interventions**
fasting
sit-ins
stay-in strike
overloading of
administration

Summary

The promotion of health often involves activities that are 'political' and involve policies of governments. This chapter has described how people and groups have tried to make governments and multi-national companies adopt health-promoting policies. Some of the lessons are:

- There may be little you can do on your own. Find people with more influence and power who will support your case.
- Try to persuade respected bodies such as professional associations and churches to pass resolutions and take up the case.
- It is always easier to ignore, discipline and attack individuals. If you are dealing with something controversial it is better to have your views coming from a *group* of people rather than named individuals who can be exposed and publicly criticized.
- It is much easier for officials to ignore criticism if no evidence is presented. So always support your case with accurate information. Include specific examples, with testimonies and photographs, of the harm that is being done by a particular policy.
- Newspapers and other media can be used to promote your case and you should be prepared to brief journalists, stage 'media events' and prepare press releases.
- Issues often have international dimensions, and involve multinational companies and international agencies. In this case you should form links with groups in other countries and international agencies. Some useful addresses are provided in Appendix C.
- If your cause is a just one, you will have the support of a network of well-wishers within your country and abroad. Don't give up!

11. Putting it into practice

By now, if you have followed the earlier chapters in this book, you should be able to determine influences on human behaviours, choose communication messages/methods and plan teaching activities. This chapter will describe how you can put everything together into a planned programme of activities and:

1. Set objectives.
2. Look at needs, research the problem, develop a strategy.
3. Monitor and evaluate your work.
4. Make a workplan and prepare a plan/project proposal.
5. Implement and manage the programme.

The planning process

Imagine that you are about to take a journey. You know where you are and have to decide where it is you want to go. Then you must decide the best way of getting to your destination. If you don't arrive at the place you wanted to go, you realise that you are lost.

Planning a health education programme is like planning a journey. Your starting-point is the present health situation, e.g. level of immunization, or sanitation, that you would like to improve to a better level, which is your 'destination'. To do this, you must decide on a *strategy* – the methods you must use to improve the situation. At the end you evaluate your programme to find out if you have reached your target – or have got lost!

When you plan your programme, you are making four sets of decisions:

- Decisions on the present situation – *where are we now?*
- Deciding desired future outcome – *where do we want to go?*
- Decisions on methods or strategy – *how will we get there?*
- Decisions on evaluation strategy – *how will we know when we get there?*

Fig. 11.1 Planning a programme is like planning a journey

207

Fig. 11.2 The planning process

A good way of finding out the present situation is to carry out a community profile or 'diagnosis' as described in Chapter 6. Setting objectives involves making decisions about how much improvement of the present situation is needed and what can be achieved with the time, money and resources available.

In earlier chapters, I showed that we can predict the likelihood of promoting a particular action through an understanding of the economic and cultural influences as well as the felt needs of the community. The amount of change you can expect to achieve will depend on the *nature of your proposed changes* (Are they simple to perform? Do they fit in with existing practices? Do they fit in with the felt needs of the community?); and *your available resources* (time, personnel and money).

You should *consider alternative methods* and their likely effectiveness before choosing the one that is most suited to your situation. In Chapter 3, guidelines were given on the likely effectiveness of different methods. A useful guide to deciding how much you can achieve is to find out how much change took place in similar settings with other programmes.

How free are you to try out new ideas? Are there any restrictions on your actions from your job description, situation, pressure from employers and the policies of your government? One important restraint is the extent to which you are able to work with fieldworkers from other departments and voluntary agencies. It will be necessary to influence economic and social factors which do not fall within the normal roles of health educators such as housing, education, agriculture, community development, employment and women's rights.

In setting targets for change you should be ambitious and try to achieve as much as possible – but also be realistic!

Aims and objectives

Aims are general statements of what the programme is trying to achieve, such as:

Health for all by the year 2000.
To improve the health of children in Chikoko District.
To increase the number of people using latrines.

Aims are not measurable and many wonder why bother to include them in documents at all! As general statements they can be useful in getting everyone to agree about a common purpose. However, more specific statements are needed when planning programmes. An 'objective' is a statement of proposed change over a fixed time period. An objective should be *measurable*. Setting measurable objectives will enable you to:

208

- let others know exactly what you are planning;
- make decisions about implementation; and
- evaluate the programme.

Another word for objective is a target. There can be much confusion in the way people use these terms. Some people use the word goal instead of aim, others use objective to describe a general statement of intention! However, it doesn't really matter what terms you use providing that you can recognize the difference between a general and a detailed measurable statement of planned activities. Make sure that you always include specific statements of proposed changes in *your* plan.

Intermediate and impact objectives

You can set objectives for the intended *outcomes* of the programme. It is also useful to set objectives for *intermediate stages* on the way to reaching your desired outcome. These are sometimes called operational – or intermediate – objectives. Later in this chapter you will see how these intermediate objectives can be displayed on a workplan and bar chart and used to monitor a programme.

outcome objectives: improvements in health
changes in behaviour
changes in knowledge, beliefs and attitudes
intermediate objectives: initial surveys
formation of organizing committee
training of key workers
field visits
broadcasting radio programmes
testing educational materials
printing publications
purchase of equipment
completion of health education activities
evaluation surveys

Writing measurable objectives

An objective for a communication should specify:

- the **intended change** in a detailed measurable form,
  e.g. acquire facts, develop decision-making ability, change beliefs, change behaviour, learn a practical skill, completion of the training programme.
- the **amount of change** above the initial baseline level,
  e.g. the percentage able to demonstrate to the interviewer the correct method for oral rehydration solution should increase from 10 to 50 per cent,
- **who** the communication should be directed at (including where they live) – often called the 'target audience',
  e.g. grandmothers in Eastern Province, adult men in Lusaka, church ministers in whole country, teachers in Chingleput District, women with one child in Yunnan Province,
- the **time scale** over which the desired change should take place,
  e.g. over the next twelve months,
- changes that are **relevant** and **realistic**.

Some problems with objectives

If objectives are so important, why are some people afraid to set them? This can be for several reasons. The present situation may be so uncertain that there is no data from which to set an initial baseline or make sensible decisions on what can be achieved. Then, the best strategy would be to plan some research and data-gathering at the start. Once data are available you can set objectives for the remaining period of the plan.

Some people feel that, if you honestly believe in community participation, it is wrong to set objectives, as these should come from the community. However, in Chapter 6 you were shown how to set objectives for *processes* within a community participation approach such as the formation of committees and reaching group decisions.

One reason for not setting objectives is that people may feel threatened by openly stating their objectives. They may feel that others will criticize them if they fail to reach the targets. It is important therefore to set objectives that are realistic for the problem you are trying to solve and the resources at your disposal. Even so, failing to reach objectives is not something to be ashamed of – provided you evaluate and find out why the activities failed and avoid those mistakes in future activities.

Research in health education and health promotion

One important reason many health education programmes fail is that the activities undertaken were planned with a poor understanding of the problem. Research involves the *systematic* collection of information (often called 'data') *to answer particular questions*. In earlier chapters you saw how important it was to understand your community and its special needs. Selection of what factors to change, choice of communication methods and content of messages should be determined from

Table 11.1 The role of research in communication programmes

Problem definition	Community surveys to determine the level of disease/trends and felt needs of the community.
Determining role of human behaviour	Surveys of community practices; research on prevention and control of disease.
Understanding influences on community behaviour	Surveys to determine influences on behaviour; sources of knowledge; role and origins of beliefs; influential persons in family and community; economic and social barriers to action.
Decisions on communication strategy	Surveys to determine communication systems in community; familiarity with and exposure to different media; characteristics of target groups; effectiveness of different media; opinion leaders that can be used in the programme.
Programme implementation	Pre-testing of messages and materials; evaluation of training; development of education methods; monitoring of progress.
Evaluation and feedback	evaluation research.

characteristics of the intended audience. Some of the areas where research can help you to plan your health education and health promotion activities are shown in Table 11.1.

Community profile

You may only need information on part of your community, e.g. out-of-school youths or the whole community. The term community profile, or 'community diagnosis', was introduced in Chapter 6 and is the process by which you systematically obtain information to understand the community in which you plan to work.

A community profile may be needed for many reasons. It can help you decide where to put your health education effort by letting you know special needs, e.g. children, elderly, families with young children, the disabled and poor. A profile might be needed to provide evidence to convince others of the need for a special programme. However, the usual reason for making a community profile is to plan a community-based health education programme.

The research process

Research is often seen as a complicated process that needs a lot of time, detailed understanding of statistics and access to facilities such as computers. As a result many people feel that they cannot do research and just base their activities on what they feel is the right approach. But, as you saw in earlier chapters, our training and background may set us apart from the community. It can be difficult for us to imagine how a young child, old person, poor villager or member of the opposite sex really feels. We can easily be mistaken if we only rely on our own judgement and do not try to find out what people really feel about these topics.

You can still obtain worthwhile information using simple research methods which do not need large amounts of time and money. Some 'rapid appraisal' methods are described below. You can find out more about research methods in Marie Therese Feurstein's excellent handbook *Partners in Evaluation* (see Appendix A).

Deciding what information to find out

Planning a piece of research involves making decisions about:

- what information is required;
- how that information should be collected to obtain a true picture of the situation and to avoid bias and errors.

A starting-point for any research is to make a list of the questions that you want to answer. In making that list you can draw from many sources. Your experience or that of other fieldworkers may suggest topics to explore. Reports of the results of other programmes may suggest issues to consider. Behavioural science concepts or particular theories may also suggest certain kinds of information, for example the checklist of questions about social influence and health beliefs on pages 30, 32 and 37. Some questions will be determined by your topic, e.g. you may have to find out how many elderly people there are in a community and where they live. The types of information to answer these questions are listed here.

FLOW CHART FOR AN EPIDEMIOLOGICAL INVESTIGATION

Lovel, H.J. (1980) Institute of Child Health, London WC1N 1EH

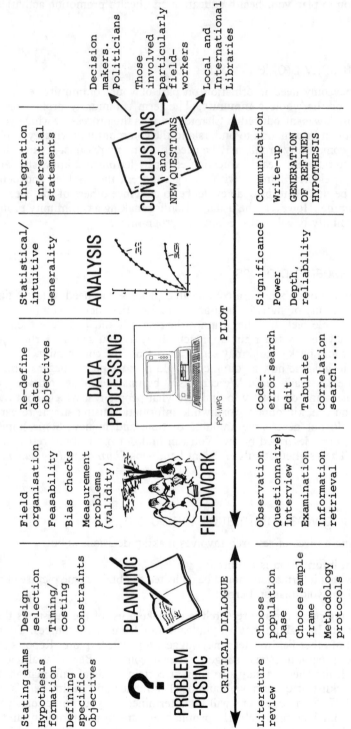

Fig. 11.3 The research process

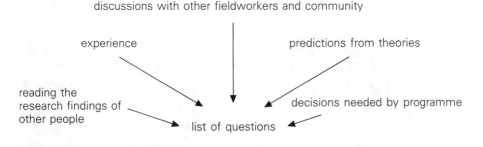

Fig. 11.4 How to generate relevant research questions

Types of information required in communication research

Basic information on the community, such as size and composition of the population, at-risk groups, income, educational level, religion, social class.
Needs of the area. Needs may be those identified by the health educator using medical criteria. They may be expressed needs that have already been put forward by the community or by the voluntary and government workers in the area or felt needs that have not yet been expressed. Many projects fail because they do not pay enough attention to expressed and felt needs of the communities.
Existing channels of communication within a community. These may be informal channels, such as neighbourhood social networks, opinion leaders, shopkeepers, tea shops, etc. or formal channels such as schools, health workers, community workers, youth leaders. Also important are details of what media are available and popular, e.g. newspapers, magazines, radio and television programmes. Find out what health information is already being conveyed through these existing channels of communication. Does it agree with or contradict your own messages? Can you mobilize these communication channels?
Influences on health behaviour. These were described in Chapter 2. Influences may operate at the individual, family, community level or higher level. They include the physical conditions of the area such as housing, the environment and the availability and quality of services such as clinics and schools; the local norms, attitudes, values and knowledge that make up the community culture; and the power structure both formal, through elected politicians and officials, and informal, through community leaders, opinion leaders and significant others.
Baseline data for evaluation Information gathered at the initial stage of making the community profile provides the baseline data to set objectives and evaluate your programme.

Deciding how to obtain the information

The data collection methods you use should provide the information you need and give a real picture of the situation. Some of the mistakes to avoid are: only believing data when it fits in with what you think is going on; people telling you what they want you to know, and not the actual truth – they may deliberately hide the truth or just find your questions confusing and difficult to answer; and

Fig. 11.5 Interviewing in Thailand

asking the views of a small group of people who do not represent the whole community. You can avoid many of these problems by following the guidelines listed here.

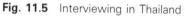

Guidelines for avoiding bias in research

- Use more than one method or source of information and then check if the information obtained from the different methods agrees – this is called 'triangulation'.
- Choose the people you talk to (your 'sample') to make sure that they are *representative* e.g. for age, sex, education, income, etc. of the group you are investigating. Don't just interview people who are easier to contact, e.g. who live nearby, come to clinics. One way of sampling the population is to make a *random* sample. For example, you could write down the names of all the people on separate sheets of paper and pick them out of a box. Another simple approach is to select every third house you come across (although in some cases that might result in biases).
- Take time to explain why you are finding out the information. People are more likely to answer you truthfully if they trust you and believe that you are going to use the information to help them. Be honest about how you will use the information and emphasize that any information provided will be confidential. It may be better to ask someone else to do the interviewing if you think that it will provide more truthful answers: for example, you can use a young person to interview another young person, a woman to interview a woman, an older person to interview an older person.

214

- Find out whether in your community there are subjects that are considered taboo and impolite to talk about. If this is the type of information you are trying to find out, you will have to consider carefully how you can ask these questions. One approach is to emphasize the confidentiality of the information.
- Avoid leading persons to answer in particular ways by the questions you ask. Explain that you really are interested in what they *themselves* think. Wherever possible, ask open questions that allow people to give frank opinions in their own words and tell you what *they* think is important.
- Involve the local communities themselves in planning the survey and doing the interviewing. This approach is called *participatory research*. This is a good way to encourage community participation and ensure that the community profile includes data that the local community sees as important (see Chapter 6).

Quantitative and qualitative research

Quantitative research methods collect specific information and facts that can be expressed as numbers. The numbers can then be treated mathematically to produce overall data for the community, e.g. the number of households with latrines, the number of children, specific knowledge about nutrition, numbers of people who hold a particular belief about the spread of AIDS. Quantitative information can be obtained through observation by looking for specific practices. Quantitative data can also be obtained from questionnaires and interviews that ask 'closed' questions – this is where people have to answer in a particular way by saying yes or no or agreeing or disagreeing with statements on a list.

open-ended question   *What do you think are the causes of diarrhoea?*
closed question: *Do you agree that diarrhoea is caused by teething?*
           Yes/no

Qualitative research methods ask 'open-ended' questions, which the respondents answer in their own words and are given freedom to expand and give their thoughts on the subject. Interviews and observation are also used to focus group discussion. Qualitative research methods can give rich insights into the local situation and people's feelings. But it is difficult to summarize the information obtained and get a complete picture of a community. Interpretation of qualitative data depends a great deal on the honesty and skill of the person doing the interviews. It is easy to introduce bias by letting your own feelings and interests influence how you interpret the data.

Qualitative research is particularly useful for 'rapid appraisals' of the situation. It is also used a great deal in helping to develop appropriate communication messages. You can find out the views of young people, test (or pre-test) media such as posters, radio programmes and get a feel for the impact of a health education programme. However, quantitative data are necessary if you have to get some idea of the size of a problem or need to convince policymakers of the need to take action.

In practice it is best to try to include a combination of qualitative and quantitative methods. One approach is to use qualitative approaches to get a 'feel' for the situation and to identify issues to lead to quantitative surveys.

Sources of data

Published sources and records and interviews with field staff

Start with existing sources such as the Census, previous surveys and records and files of agencies operating in the area. It is surprising how much useful information can be obtained from the most unlikely sources such as government reports, minutes of meetings and newspaper reports. However, much of the available information can be of poor quality, irrelevant and out of date. Health data from clinics and hospital data can give a useful picture of the local situation but only represent cases where people have come for treatment. They will miss out people who have been treated at home or taken to private or traditional healers.

Look out for field staff from health and other services who have worked in the community and can give you the benefit of their experience. Try to speak to some of them and see if they agree with each other and with what members of the community themselves say.

Interviews in the community

The next stage of data collection is to go to the area and meet the people that live and work there. But be careful – surveys can be expensive and time-consuming and arouse expectations of action that you may not be able to fulfil.

It is often more efficient to interview informally members of the community and workers in various government and voluntary organizations – the 'key informants'. This provides information about the area and is an opportunity to introduce yourself and your health education interests. Give careful thought to whom you can interview to get a balanced and true picture. Your informants might give different and contradictory responses. But even these differences can tell you a great deal, as it is important to understand the conflicts and tensions within the community. Leaving out a key person may also cause problems later if they feel that their views are being ignored!

Focused group discussions

These are discussions with groups of people in the community carried out in a systematic way to provide information on a topic. Groups of people sharing the same characteristics are brought together. A group discussion is guided by questions asked by the interviewer. These should be open-ended and designed to make people respond and discuss. You should try to limit your own involvement to that of a facilitator. You should encourage discussion *between* the group members so you can observe the language used and feelings of the group.

Observation

Another way to get to know a community is 'street work' or observation. This involves casual observations and informal conversations with residents of the area on doorsteps, in public places, shops, etc. It is also possible to have 'structured' observation with a checklist of points to look out for so that the observation is carried out in a systematic way – see the list here for an example of an observational checklist.

Health practices: observational checklist developed for *Mtu Ni Afya* radio health education project in Tanzania

1. Is there vegetation growing near the house?
2. Are there depressions, holes, or receptacles of any kind near the house that could hold stagnant water?
3. Is there mosquito netting over the bed(s) in the bedroom(s)?
4. Is there mosquito netting on the windows?
5. Is there a latrine that meets *Mtu Ni Afya* standards?
6. Does the latrine have a cover?
7. Is the latrine being used?
8. Is the courtyard around the house free of rubbish?
9. Are there any animal faeces near the house?
10. Are there any rats, other vermin or other pests visible in or around the house?
11. Does the house have any windows?
12. Are there a lot of flies in or around the house?

Action-research approaches

You can find out the feelings of the community by carrying out some health education and asking for comments and feedback. For example you can ask people's opinions about a leaflet, poster or show a film. You might try setting up an advice-stall and monitor what requests for information come from the community.

Planning a survey

Surveys can use any of the data collection methods described above on all, or a sample, of the people in a community. Before doing a full-scale survey of a community it is better first to carry out a small-scale 'pilot' such as interviews and focus group discussions so you already have an idea of the important topics to include and try out the questions. In planning your survey, you can follow the steps in Figure 11.3 and the list of 'Questions to ask'.

Questions to ask in planning community health surveys

Stage 1: Define aims and scope of the study
Why do you need to undertake the survey? What are the needs and problems to be investigated? How will you use the information obtained? Can the information be obtained in any other way?

Stage 2: Decide upon the information requirements
What information is required to deal with the community's needs and problems?
What information is needed for proposing a solution or for allocating resources to the health and community needs?
What do the local fieldworkers feel you should include in the survey?
What do the community feel you should include in the survey?
If funds are limited, what are the most important questions to ask?

Stage 3: Find out whether the required information is already available
Has a survey already been carried out in the community that might contain useful information? Are there any books or published reports that deal with a similar need in other communities, at a regional or at a national level?

Stage 4: Assess whether the survey can succeed
Will a survey provide the information you need?
Are there sufficient resources (money, field staff) and time to carry out the survey?

Stage 5: Making decisions on data-collection, sampling and implementation
How will the data be collected – observation, interviews, focus group discussions? If using observation, what will you include in the checklist? If asking questions, what wording will you use and how will you test the questions to make sure they are understood and acceptable?
How are the communities and people in the sample to be selected? How many are to be included? How long will each interview/observation visit take?
When will the data collection take place – time of day, day of week, season? How long will the survey take to complete?
Who will you use to carry out the interviewing? Can you involve local field workers, volunteers or members of the community? Will they need training?
What arrangements are needed to get the interviewers to the field?
How are you going to involve the community in your survey?
How much time is needed to complete all the fieldwork including visiting and interviewing?
How will you analyze and present the data?

Stage 6: Estimating the cost of the survey and preparing a budget
How much will it cost to undertake the survey including transport, staffing and other help?
Are there non-essential questions that can be left out of the survey to reduce the cost? Could the number of people or geographical area of the sample be reduced?

Evaluation

The systematic and scientific process determining the extent to which an action or set of actions were successful in the achievement of pre-determined objectives. It involves measurement of adequacy, effectiveness and efficiency of health services.

WHO (1969)

We evaluate to aid future planning and to improve programmes, to increase our understanding of health education practice, to add to the body of knowledge upon which our work is based. We evaluate to achieve operational efficiency and, related to this, to obtain data that permit interpretation of programme effectiveness so as to obtain administrative support, community support and even functional support. We evaluate for reasons associated with motivation – to give staff and volunteers satisfaction, and a sense of success. To give priority to these purposes ... we evaluate primarily to study the effects of practice so that we can turn our findings back into practice and improve it and, at the same time, strengthen the scientific basis of practice in health education.

Beryl Roberts (1962).

We evaluate communication and health education programmes for many reasons. The most important reason is to learn from our experiences and to improve our methods. The health education methods described in this book have been developed in many different countries and may not work in other situations. You will need to find out what will work in *your own* setting. Health education can only develop as a serious discipline if we build up experience from evaluated programmes.

But there are other important reasons: you may need to evaluate your programmes to show that you are doing your job properly; you may need to justify the money you have received from a funding body; people around you may not believe that health education works and you may need to convince them to give you their support. So evaluations are done for many reasons – some open and others hidden. You will need to decide at the outset *why* you are evaluating your programme and *who* the evaluation is intended for. Some important terms used in evaluation are:

- **effectiveness** – whether or not a programme achieves its stated objectives, i.e. did it work?
- **efficiency** – the amount of effort in terms of time, manpower, resources and money required to reach the objectives – was it worth the effort?
- **formative evaluation** – 'monitoring' progress during the programme involving measurement of intermediate objectives, i.e. what have we achieved so far?
- **summative evaluation** – measurement of impact or change at the end of the programme, i.e. have we achieved our objectives?

So evaluation involves showing that:

- **change** has taken place;
- the change took place as a **result** of the programme;
- the amount of **effort** required to produce the change was worthwhile.

So, evaluating your health education involves making some important decisions. What changes should you measure? How should you measure those changes? How can you prove that the changes took place as a result of the programme? Decisions about what changes to measure and how to measure them are really decisions about what should be your *objectives*. These were discussed in an earlier section of this chapter.

Most people would agree that it is important in evaluation to show that change has taken place. But the need to show that change took place as a result of your programme is less obvious. Consider the following situations where external factors had an influence on a programme:

1. An increase in immunization takes place because a government minister makes a broadcast in the middle of your field campaign.
2. An influential person returns from the city and starts to encourage villagers where you are doing your sanitation programme.
3. In the middle of your AIDS education campaign a famous film star dies of AIDS and this leads to more people adopting safer sex.
4. Diarrhoea rates drop during the four months of the programme – but this would have taken place anyway because of the normal seasonal fall after the rainy season.

Does it really matter that other factors helped your programme? Perhaps not. But what if your programme was an experimental pilot project testing out a new approach that you want to repeat elsewhere? You would have to make certain that the improvements made really had come about because of your new methods and not for other reasons. Otherwise money and effort would be wasted repeating methods that do not actually work!

One reason evaluation is difficult is that it is often only at the end of a programme that thought is given to how the programme should be evaluated. In fact, you should plan at the beginning how you will evaluate your work.

Communication stages and evaluation

It is always best to anticipate problems by 'pre-testing' communications with samples of the intended audience before you begin your main activities. However it is still important to evaluate the programme at the end to find out how effective you have been. In Chapter 3 you saw how communications can fail at many stages from reaching the sense organs up to changing health. Communication failure can take place at each of the six stages. If you ask the following questions and find out at which stage a failure in communication took place, you can correct the fault and improve the programme.

Questions to ask when evaluating communication activities

Were the communication activities carried out?
How many radio programmes were broadcast; talks/training sessions given; community meetings held; leaflets distributed; posters put up?
Did the intended audience come across the message?
How many people saw the posters, were able to receive the radio broadcasts, come to the talks, passed by the exhibition?
Did the intended audience pay attention to the communication?
What was the 'coverage' of the programme – how many people saw the poster, listened to the radio programme, stopped to look at the exhibition, were paying attention at the meeting?
Did the intended audience understand the messages?
How many people could correctly repeat back the messages in the posters, radio programmes, talks, meetings?
Did it convince the audience?
How many people accepted and believed the message?
Did it result in a change in behaviour?
How many people changed their behaviour as a result of the communication?
Did it lead to improvements in health?
How many people's health improved as a result of the programme?
What changes in level of disease incidence/prevalence took place?

You should be realistic over what changes to look for in your evaluation. Changes in knowledge, understanding, awareness and belief might take place soon after the communication. However, changes in behaviour and health usually take longer to achieve. It is a good idea to carry out a *short-term evaluation* fairly soon after the activity and a *follow-up evaluation* afterwards to look for long-term changes.

Showing that change took place because of your programme

If the objectives have been clearly defined at the outset, it is not usually difficult to show that change has taken place in your community. However, it is much more difficult to show that it took place *because of your own efforts* and not because of another reason. There are two ways of showing that change was caused by your own efforts (this is called proving 'causality'): see Figure 11.6.

220

1. Using controls

measure baseline
at the beginning
programme
– 'pre-test'
for test group and
control group

test group receives education

control group does not
receive education

measure levels
at the end of the

– 'post-test'

2. Indirect evaluation without a control

measure baseline ——→ give education ——→ measure levels at
at the beginning of the group   end, ask questions
                                              to find out why people
                                              changed and find out if it was
                                              because of your effort

Fig. 11.6 Two approaches to evaluation

Using controls

You can set up another group, e.g. another classroom, group of mothers, another village as a 'control' who do not receive the education. The two groups should be as close as possible in age, education and income. If the group that received your educational programme achieves a better performance than the control group, this will provide strong evidence for the success of your communication activities.

Indirect method without controls

If it is not possible to set up a control group you will have to use an indirect method for excluding other reasons for any changes. You could look carefully at what has taken place – could there be any other possible explanation for the changes that took place? You could interview samples of the community and ask them why they changed their behaviour – was it because of your activities or were there other reasons that you were not aware of?

Participatory evaluation

In Chapter 6 the idea of participatory evaluation was introduced. Involvement of the community in evaluation helps to create a bond of trust with the community: you can find out their feelings about the benefits and weaknesses of your activities; you can draw on their experiences and insights on what has happened; evaluation becomes a learning process and the community is able to reflect on its experiences and plan future activities. Guidelines on evaluation are given overleaf.

- Decide at the beginning of a programme how you are going to evaluate it.
- Prepare a set of realistic, achievable and measurable indicators for success. Consult your employers, funding bodies and the community when you decide on your objectives.
- Wherever possible, set up control groups who do not receive the education. If controls are not possible, collect data that will help you to show that it was your efforts that led to improvements.
- Look for changes in the short term as well as long term. Find out if any benefits are long-lasting.
- Don't limit yourself to finding out if you have reached your objectives – look out for any unplanned benefits or unexpected problems.
- Look out for ways of involving the target groups in all the stages of the evaluation process including setting objectives, collecting data, judging outcomes and deciding on future activities.
- Learn from your failures as well as your successes. Find out why programmes succeeded or failed and what lessons can be drawn for the future.
- Share your successes or failures with others. Tell others about what you have been doing, circulate any reports and look out for newsletters and journals to which you can send articles.

Preparing a workplan

Even if your work only involves a few simple activities, it is still worthwhile planning your time. This helps you to use your time efficiently, spread your workload, anticipate needs and avoids last-minute panic. A simple workplan is to write intended activities on a calendar and circle important days. You can buy or draw for yourself a 'year planner'. This is a large sheet with a square for each day of the year on which you can write key activities using colours to show particular tasks.

Other useful approaches are to set out your objectives as a table or a 'bar chart' (sometimes called 'Gannt' chart) for a particular programme on which you can show dates for completing planned activities (see Figure 11.7 and the communication strategy in Figure 3.16). You can also set out a workplan as a table that sets out, for each planned activity the person responsible for carrying out the activity, the date for completion, and how you will measure achievement and cost.

Plan documents and project proposals

When you are setting up a special programme with a range of activities over a period of time and a series of objectives, it is useful to write them into a *plan document*.

You may need a written plan to seek approval from your employers that you should spend time on the activity and that you need money for equipment, transport and living expenses. However, a written plan is useful for other reasons: it makes sure that everyone is aware of what will be taking place and supports

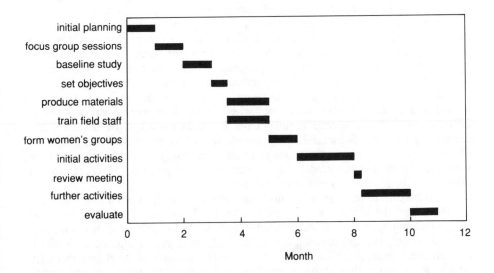

Women's Nutrition Project
Schedule of activities

Sample workplan for a 'Women's Nutrition Project'

Activities	Responsible person	Month	Indicators of achievement	Cost (US$)
1. Hold a two day workshop to orient staff on women's nutrition project.	programme manager	Jan. 1993	completed workshop	1 000
2. Conduct 8 focus group interviews with women in the target community.	research officer, health education officer	Feb.	report on focus group interviews and recommendations	3 000
3. Complete baseline study of nutrition beliefs and practices of 400 households.	research officer, nutrition field staff	March	completed interviews and data analysis report on baseline study	20 000
4. Produce set of measurable objectives for programme based on the data from baseline study.	programme manager chief nutrition officer	April	Document distributed with specific measurable objectives	300
5. Develop, pre-test and print training handbook and resource book for women on weaning foods.	health education officer artist	May	copies of training handbook and leaflet printed and ready for distribution.	40 000

Fig. 11.7 Workplan and bar chart: Women's Nutrition Project, schedule of activities

the proposed activities; it saves much time explaining to others what will actually take place; it is also a good way of allowing others to comment and make suggestions on how your plans can be improved; getting a plan approved saves time later as you will not need to obtain clearance for each separate activity.

A *project proposal* is a document outlining proposed activities and seeking permission and/or funds to proceed. A *plan* is the document that specifies what is actually going to happen. Often the same document meets both needs: before it is approved, the document is a proposal; after approval, the document is modified to take into account any suggested changes and called 'the plan'.

If you are preparing a proposal to go to a funding agency for approval it is a good idea to find out from that agency whether they have any special procedures. Often a sponsor has special requirements for information to be included in a request for funding. Sometimes they provide special forms to write the proposals. Sponsors can have different interests and these can change over time. For example, some may insist that you emphasize community participation or reaching women, others may be mainly interested in children.

It is helpful to meet people who have been successful in obtaining funds and ask them how they have done it. You can try to obtain copies of recent proposals that have been approved. Another useful approach is to have an informal meeting with someone from the funding agency to find out if your proposed activities fit in with their interests. You could write a short summary of what you intend to do and ask them if they think it worth your going to the trouble of preparing a detailed proposal.

If the activity you are undertaking is short and will be completed in a few days, your project proposal need only be a few pages. If your activities cover a longer period, involve large expenses and cooperation of many bodies, your document will be longer. Guidelines for preparing a project proposal are given below. Even if you do not have to produce a written plan, it is a good idea to apply these steps. They will help you to use your time in a way that is both effective and efficient.

Preparing a project proposal

1. ***Title for the programme.*** The title of the project should describe the purpose of the project.
2. ***Summary of plan.*** Many people will not have time to read your whole plan so it is important to have a one-page summary at the beginning that lists details of proposed activities, objectives, management and budget. This should contain section or page references to the parts of the plan they deal with.
3. ***Table of contents.*** This should help the readers find any section of the document that they want.
4. ***Statement of need or of the problem to be tackled.*** The problem should be described using supporting data wherever possible. The population at risk should be described, including the size of the problem, seriousness of impact on the community, whether the problem is getting worse, data on the community and the number of people who need to be reached.

   The communication and health education problem needs to be defined: this should include an analysis of the current situation and shortfalls in health, scope for prevention of disability and premature death and the identification of any health-related behaviours that may need to be changed.

5. *Mechanisms for obtaining participation of all groups.* This section should describe how you propose to involve all the key groups in the various stages of your programme, including defining problems, setting objectives, planning, implementation and evaluation. These key groups are the community, relevant local groups and fieldworkers in health and other services.

6. *Specification of your objectives.* In this section you should list your objectives and give reasons why each one has been selected. The objectives should be appropriate to the problem you have defined and should be achievable within the time-scale you have specified.

7. *Analysis of factors influencing achievement of objectives and identification of strategies including educational methods.* You should:
   - describe the positive and negative forces affecting the problem, drawing on behavioural models (see Chapter 2), lessons learned from previous research and previous experiences.
   - identify any enabling factors that might require supportive economic measures and improvements in health services.
   - list target groups and beliefs that you are seeking to influence.
   - outline your communication methods, messages and who is to carry out the communication; give reasons for your choice, e.g. feasibility, cost, suitability to the target group and desired change. (See Chapter 3.)

8. *Management of the activities.* Your plan should explain how you will manage your proposed activities. It is important to say who will be responsible for each activity and describe the nature of any steering group or management committee. A good way of showing this is to include an organization diagram or 'organogram' that shows the different individuals and groups involved and the lines of responsibility and communication. It is also helpful to describe the role key persons can play in the programme and provide job specifications. As described in Chapter 4, these job specifications can also be used to explain training needs.

9. *Resources and budget.* This part of the plan should consider the needs for money, personnel, facilities, equipment and supplies. The budget should be enough to carry out the proposed tasks. You should allow for increases in prices of goods and have a contingency of at least 10 per cent to cover unforeseen costs. There should be a description of how the funds will be managed, including book-keeping, issuing of petty cash and payment of bills.

10. *Timetable/workplan.* This part of the plan sets out the timescale for achieving the planned activities such as training, materials production and surveys. The best way to show the sequence of activities is a bar chart (see Figure 11.7).

11. *Evaluation.* This section describes how you will monitor and evaluate the effectiveness and efficiency of the programme. You should explain how you will obtain reliable and valid data to measure achievement of objectives, completion of the different planned activities; use of resources and spending of budgeted funds; unforeseen benefits and disadvantages; community as well as other interested groups' views on the value of the programme. You should provide a list of the indicators of effectiveness that you will be using.

Managing the programme

This will involve answering the following questions.

- How will you coordinate and support the activities of the different field staff and organisations taking part and involve them in decisions on future activities?

- How will you communicate new information, skills and changes of policy to all involved?
- How will you ensure that the findings from any monitoring and research activities are acted upon as quickly as possible?
- How will you maintain the community participation throughout the programme?

A common problem in health education is that fieldworkers give different and conflicting advice, and workers and the community become confused as to what exactly they should do. So you must ensure that everyone is briefed to give the correct information.

At the outset of the programme it is a good idea to run a training workshop to brief those involved, provide any necessary information and give an opportunity to learn any new communication skills.

You will need to maintain the momentum and enthusiasm of your programme. People are more likely to support your programme and put effort into activities if they think that you are taking an interest in what they are doing and are supporting them with advice and resources.

One way to keep in touch is to arrange a regular schedule of visits to different groups. However, the amount of travelling can be reduced if you bring people together for regular meetings to introduce new ideas, review progress and decide future actions. You can carry out your meetings in an effective way by applying the principles of group dynamics that were outlined in Chapter 5.

In addition to these meetings with field staff you will need to set up meetings once or twice a year with your employers, senior persons in the various agencies participating in the project and the funding body. This formal management group would review the progress, receive reports and financial statements.

Setting up a resource centre

It is important to keep up-to-date with new developments yourself and to find ways of passing on information to others. One approach is to build up a small resource collection of newsletters as well as any books or teaching materials you have. You can display them in a room so that others can see them. Details are provided at the end of this book of a range of useful books that are available by mail order from Teaching Aids at Low Cost who also provide slide sets and other teaching materials. In Appendix B, I have included addresses of some free newsletters providing updates on a range of health topics. You should include in your project budget the cost of a resource collection of books. This is an expenditure that most sponsors will support. If you do build up a resource collection, you should distribute a catalogue to let others know what you have, and develop a simple system for lending them out and making sure that they are returned.

Another good way of keeping in touch with others in your programme is through a regular newsletter. This can be produced simply with information on health topics and current activities. Field staff and the community can contribute through letters and articles and you can answer any questions. You can also include extracts from international newsletters on health topics.

Educational materials such as leaflets, posters and visual aids can be kept in your resource centre for distribution to others. You should take care to store them in a dry and clean place so they do not get damaged. You will have to set up a system for distributing posters and educational materials to the various groups in your project.

Summary

In this chapter I have given some practical guidelines on how you can plan, manage and evaluate your communication programmes.

1. You should decide your objectives and how you will evaluate the programme at the beginning.
2. It is helpful to set out your procedures for management, community participation, monitoring and evaluation in a written plan.
3. Good communication is essential to management.
4. You should share your successes and failures with others so that the lessons learned will lead to better programmes. Why not send descriptions of your activities to the newsletters and journals listed in Appendix B?

Appendix A A basic reading list

1. Introducing health education and health promotion

A. General health issues

Burgers, L. *et al.* (1988) *Hygiene Education in Water Supply and Sanitation Programmes*. IRC International Reference Centre for Community Water Supply and Sanitation Programmes, PO Box 93190, 2509 AD The Hague, Netherlands.

Brown, R. C., Brown, J. E. (1987) *The Family Planning Clinic in Africa*. Macmillan, London.

Gordon, G. and Klouda, A. (1988) *Talking AIDS – A guide for community workers*. Macmillan, London.

Harpham, T. *et al.* (1988) *In the Shadow of the City – Community health and the urban poor*. Oxford University Press, Oxford.

Hubley, J. H. (1989) *The AIDS Handbook – An introduction to AIDS and HIV*. Macmillan, London.

King, F. Savage and Burgess, A. (1992) *Nutrition for Developing Countries*. Oxford University Press, Oxford.

Morley, D. and Lovel, H. (1986) *My Name is Today. An illustrated discussion of child health, society and poverty in less developed countries*. Macmillan, London.

Morley, D. and Woodland, M. (1979) *See How They Grow. Monitoring child growth for appropriate health care in developing countries*. Macmillan Tropical Community Health Manual, Macmillan, London.

Morley, D. *et al.* (1983) *Practising Health for All*. Oxford University Press, Oxford.

Pierre, B. *et al.* (1983) *Alcoholism*. Bureau for the Study and Research for the Promotion of Health, PO Box 1800 Kangu-Mayombe, Republic of Zaire.

Sabatier, R. (1987) *AIDS and the Third World – The Panos Dossier*. Panos Institute, London.

Sanders, D. (1985) *The Struggle for Health – Medicine and the politics of underdevelopment*.

UNICEF, WHO and UNESCO (n.d.) *Facts For Life*. UNICEF, New York.

UNICEF (1984 and subsequent years) *The State of the World's Children Reports*. UNICEF, New York.

Werner, D. *Disabled Village Children – A guide for community health workers, rehabilitation workers and families*. Hesperion Foundation, Palo Alto, California.

WHO/SEARO (1985) *Achieving Success in Community Water Supply and Sanitation Projects*. WHO South East Asia Regional Papers No. 9, WHO, New Delhi.

WHO/UNICEF (1980) *Primary Health Care. Report of the International conference on primary health care – Alma Ata Declaration*. WHO, Geneva.

B. Books on health education and health promotion

American Society of Public Health (1975) 'Making Health Education Work', *American Journal of Public Health* supplement 65.

Favin, M.*et al.* (1986) *Health Education – Information for action issue paper.* World Federation of Public Health Association, Geneva.

Green, L. W. *et al.* (1980) *Health Education Planning – A diagnostic approach.* Mayfield, Palo Alto, California.

WHO (1988) *Education for Health – Manual on health education in primary health care.* WHO, Geneva.

2. Understanding human behaviour

Ajzen, I. and Fishbein, M. (1980) *Understanding Attitudes and Predicting Social Behaviour.* Prentice Hall, New Jersey.

Foster, E. M. and Anderson, B. G. (1978) *Medical Anthropology.* J. Wiley & Sons, New York.

Paul, B. D. (1955) *Health, Culture and the Community. Case studies of public reactions to public health programmes.* Russell Sage Foundation, New York.

3. An introduction to communication

Bertrand, J. T. (1978) *Communication Pretesting.* Media Monograph 6, Communication and Family Study Centre, Chicago.

National Institute of Health (1984) *Pretesting in Health Communications.* NIH Publication.

Rasmuson, M. R. *et al.* (1988) *Communication for Child Survival.* Healthcom, Academy for Educational Development, Washington, DC.

UNICEF (1976) *Communicating with Pictures in Nepal* – Report of a study by NDS and UNICEF. UNICEF, PO Box 1187, Kathmandu, Nepal.

Rogers, E. (1983) *Diffusion of Innovations.* The Free Press, New York.

Rogers, E. M. and Shoemaker (1971) *Communications of Innovations – A cross-cultural approach.* Free Press, New York.

UNICEF (n.d.) *Rethinking Visual Literacy – Helping pre-literates learn.* UNICEF, Nepal.

WHO (1987) *Communication – A guide for managers of national diarrhoeal disease control programmes: planning, management and appraisal of communication activities.* Diarrhoeal Disease Control Programme, WHO, Geneva.

4. The effective teacher

Abbatt, F. and McMahon, R. (1985) *Teaching Health Care Workers – a practical guide.* Macmillan, London.

Fetter, K. A. *et al.* (1987) *Teaching and Learning with Visual Aids. A resource manual for community health workers, health training and family planning workers in Africa and the Middle East.* Educational Materials Unit, Programme for International Training in Community Health (INTRAH), Univiversity of North Carolina Press and Macmillan, Chapel Hill and London.

Guilbert, J. J. (1977) *Educational Handbook for Health Personnel.* WHO Offset Publication no. 35, WHO, Geneva.

Jenkins, J. (1981) *Materials for Learning. How to teach adults at a distance.* Routledge & Kegan Paul, London.

Johnstone, M. and Rifkin, S. (1989) *Health Care Together. Training exercises for health workers in community-based programmes.* Macmillan, London.

Keehn, M. (1982) *Bridging the Gap: A participatory approach to health and nutrition education.* Save the Children, 54 Wilton Road, Westport, Connecticut 06880, USA.

230

Werner, D. and Bower, B. (1982) *Helping Health Workers Learn*. Hesperion Foundation, Palo Alto, California.

5. Face-to-face

Unfortunately there are few suitable books to recommend on this with a content relevant to experiences in developing countries – maybe you should write one!

6. Working with communities

Freire, P. (1972) *Pedagogy of the Oppressed*. Penguin Books, Harmondsworth.

Kindervatter, S. (1979) *Non-formal Education as an Empowering Process*. Centre for International Education, Amherst, Massachussetts.

Martin, P. A. (1983) *Community Participation in Primary Health Care*. American Public Health Association International Health Programme, Washington.

PAHO (1984) *Community Participation in Health and Development in the Americas – An analysis of selected case studies*. PAHO Scientific Publication no. 473, Pan American Health Organization, 525 Twenty-third Street N.W., Washington, DC.

Henderson P. and Thomas D. N. (1979) *Skills in Neighbourhood Work*. Allen & Unwin, London.

Peace Corps (1978) *Community Health Education in Developing Countries – Getting started*. Peace Corps Information Collection and Exchange Programme and Training Journal Manual No. 8, US Peace Corps.

Van Wijk-Sijbesma, C. (1981) *Participation and Education in Community Water Supply and Sanitation Programmes – A literature review*. International Reference Centre for Community Water Supply and Sanitation Programmes, PO Box 93190, 2509 AD The Hague, Netherlands.

7. Communication – the people's way!

Byram, M. L. (1985) *Theatre-for-Development – A guide for training*. Centre for International Education, Amherst, Mass.

Gordon, G. and S. (1986) *Puppets for Better Health*. Macmillan, London.

Hilton, D. (1980) *Health Teaching for West Africa – Stories, drama and song*. MAP International, Illinois.

8. Using media

Church, C. A. and Geller, J. (1989) *Lights, Camera! Action! Promoting family planning with TV, video and film*. Population Reports Series J, No. 38. Baltimore, Johns Hopkins University, Population Information Program.

Colle, R. D. (1979) *The Communication Factor in Health and Nutrition Programmes. A case study and guidelines for action*. Dept of Communication Arts, Cornell University, New York.

Crowley, D., Etherington, A,, Kidd, R. and Roewendahl, P. R. (1978) *Radio Learning Group Manual*. Friedrich Ebert Stiftung, Godesberger Allee 149, 5300 Bonn 2, Germany.

Gilluly, R. H. and Moore, S. H. (1986) *Radio – Spreading the word on family planning*. Population Reports Series J, No. 32. Baltimore, Johns Hopkins University, Population Information Program.

Jenkins, J. (1983) *Mass Media for Health Education*. IEC Broadsheets on Distance Learning no. 18, International Extension College, Cambridge.

Keating, R. (1977) *Grass Roots Radio – A Manual for fieldworkers in family planning and other areas of social and economic development.* International Planned Parenthood, London.

Sweeny, W. O. (1982) *Using Radio – Primary Health Care Issues*, American Public Health Association, Washington, DC.

Weeks, D. (1976) *The Photo-novel – A tool for development.* US Peace Corps Programme and Training Manual Series, Washington, DC.

9. Working with children and young people

Aarons, A. *et al.* (1979) *Child-to-Child.* Macmillan, London.

Carlisle, J. (1988) *Toys for Fun – A book of toys for pre-school children.* Macmillan, London.

Hawes, H. (1988) *Child-To-Child – Another path to learning.* Unesco Institute for Education, Hamburg.

IRC (1988) *Water Supply and Sanitation in Primary School Education in Developing Countries.* IRC International Water and Sanitation Centre, The Hague, The Netherlands.

Morley, D. *et al.* (1984) *Mobilizing Education to Reinforce Primary Health Care.* Notes Comments {Child, family, community} Digest no. X, UNESCO, Paris.

Young, B. and Durston, S. (1987) *Primary Health Education.* Longman, Harlow.

10. Politics and health

Dinham, B. and Hines, C. (1983) *Agribusiness in Africa.* Earth Resources Research Publication, 258 Pentonville Road, London N1 9JX.

Hansson, O. (1988) *Inside CIBA-GEIGY.* IOCU, International Organisation of Consumer Unions, Penang/The Hague/Montevideo.

Melrose, D. (1982) *Bitter Pills – Medicines and the Third World poor.* Oxfam, Oxford.

Muller, M. (1982) *The Health of Nations – A north–south investigation.* Faber & Faber, London.

Palmer, G. (1988) *The Politics of Breastfeeding.* Pandora, London.

Raw, M. *et al.* (1990) *Clearing the Air – A guide for action on tobacco.* WHO Regional Office for Europe and British Medical Association, Tavistock Square, London.

Taylor, P. (1984) *The Smoke Ring – Tobacco, money and international politics.* Sphere Books, London.

11. Putting it into practice

Amonoo-Lartson, R. *et al.* (1984) *District Health Care – Challenges for planning, organisation and evaluation in developing countries.* Macmillan, London.

Debus, M. Porter/Novelli, (n.d.) *Handbook for Excellence in Focus Group Research.* Academy for Educational Development, Washington, DC.

Feuerstein, M. T. (1986) *Partners in Evaluation – Evaluating community development and community programmes with participants.* Macmillan, London.

Janovsky, K. (n.d.) *Project formulation and proposal writing.* WHO/EDUC/87.187, WHO, Geneva.

Mager, R. F. (1962) *Preparing instructional objectives.* Pitman, Belmont, California.

Perret, H. (1984) *Monitoring and Evaluation of Communication Support Activities in Low-cost Sanitation Projects.* Technology Advisory Group, World Bank, Washington.

WHO (1981) *Health Programme Evaluation – Guiding principles.* WHO, Geneva.

Appendix B Newsletters relevant to health education

Newsletter marked * are supplied free to persons from developing countries; others are available on subscription and you should write for a sample copy and their current rates.

AIDS Action * Quarterly from ARHTAG, 1 London Bridge St, London SE1 9SG, UK.

AIDS Health Promotion Exchange * Quarterly from Global Programme on AIDS, World Health Organisation, 1211 Geneva 27, Switzerland.

ARI News. * ARHTAG, 1 London Bridge St, London SE1 9SG, UK. 'An international forum for the exchange of news and views on acute respiratory infections'.

Community Eye Health. * International Centre for Eye Health, Institute for Opthalmology, 27–29 Cayton Street, London EC1V 9EJ.

Contact. * Christian Medical Commission, World Council of Churches, 150 Route de Ferney, 1211 Geneva 20, Switzerland. (Primary health care.)

Diarrhoea Dialogue. * ARHTAG, 1 London Bridge St, London SE1 9SG, UK.

Environmental Health. * WHO Newsletter on Environmental Health, World Health Organization, 1211 Geneva 27, Switzerland.

Essential Drugs Monitor. * WHO Action Programme on Essential Drugs and Vaccines, World Health Organization, 1211 Geneva 27, Switzerland.

Glimpse. * International Centre for Diarrhoeal Disease Research, GPO Box 128, Dacca-2, Bangladesh. (Diarrhoea; water; sanitation.)

Health Action. PB 2153, 157/6 Staff Road, Gunrock Enclave, Secundarabad 500 003, Andra Pradesh, India.

Health Education Research. Oxford University Press, Pinkhill House, Southfield Road, Eynsham, Oxford OX8 1JJ, UK.

Health for the Millions. Voluntary Health Association of India, 40 Qtab Institutional Area, South of IIT, New Delhi-110016, India.

Hygie (magazine of the International Union of Health Education). 9 Rue Newton, 75116, Paris, France.

International Quarterly of Community Health Education. Baywood Publishing Company Inc., 120 Marine St, PO Box D, Farmingdale, New York 11735, USA.

International Family Planning Perspectives. * Alan Guttmacher Institute, 111 Fifth Avenue, New York, NY 10003, USA.

IPPF Medical Bulletin. * International Planned Parenthood Federation, PO Box 759, Inner Circle, Regent's Park, London NW1 4NQ, UK.

IRC Bulletin. * WHO Int. Reference Centre for Community Water Supply, PO Box 550, 2280 HM Rijswijk, The Hague, Netherlands.

IRCWD News. * WHO International Reference Centre for Wastes Disposal, Uberlandstrasse 133, CH-8600 Duebendorf, Switzerland.

Mother and Children. * American Public Health Association, 1015 15th St NW, Washington DC 20005, USA. (Health, nutrition and MCH.)

Notes Comments Series. * Unit for Cooperation with UNICEF and WFP, UNESCO, 7 Place de Fontenoy, 75700 Paris, France. (Pre-school, and school health education.)

Population Reports. * Population Information Programme, Johns Hopkins School of Hygiene and Public Health, Johns Hopkins University, 62 North Broadway, Baltimore, Maryland 21205, USA. (Family planning communication.)

SEARB Bulletin. Newsletter of the South East Asia Regional Bureau of the International Union of Health Education, 6, VR Road, Madhavanagar, Bangalore-56700 001, India.

Waterlines. Intermediate Technology Publications Ltd, 103-105 Southampton Row, London WC1B 4HH, UK. (Water and sanitation.)

World AIDS. * Panos Institute, 8 Alfred Place, London WC1EB 7EB, UK.

World Health Forum. World Health Organization, 1211 Geneva, Switzerland. (Health; nutrition; health policy; details of WHO publications.)

Appendix C Useful addresses

(See also the addresses of the agencies publishing the newsletters/journals described in the previous section.)

Academy for Educational Development, 1255 23rd Street, NW, Washington, DC 20037, USA.

Action on Smoking and Health, 5–11 Mortimer Street, London W1N 7RH, UK.

African Medical and Research Foundation (AMREF), Wilson Airport, PO Box 30125, Nairobi, Kenya.

Appropriate Health Technology Action Group, (ARHTAG), 1 London Bridge Street, London SE1 9SG, UK.

Centre for Communication Programmes, Johns Hopkins School of Hygiene and Public Health, Johns Hopkins University, 62 North Broadway, Baltimore, Maryland 21205, USA.

Centre de Formation pour la Promotion de la Santé, B.P. 1800, Kangu, Mayumbe, Zaire.

Child-to-Child Programme, c/o Institute of Child Health, 30 Guildford Street, London WC1 1EH.

Educators for Rational Drug Use (ERDU), The ERDU Coordinator, IOCU Regional Office for Asia and the Pacific, PO Box 1045, 10830, Penang, Malaysia.

Health Action International-Europe, J. Van Lennepkade 334-T, 1053 NJ Amsterdam, The Netherlands.

International Baby Foods Action Network, IBFAN, c/o GIFA, C.P. 157, 1211 Geneva 19, Switzerland.

International Organization of Consumers Unions (IOCU), PO Box 1045, 10830, Penang, Malaysia.

International Confederation of Free Trade Unions, 37–41, Rue Montagne aux Herbed Potagères, B-1000, Brussels, Belgium.

International Reference Centre for Community Water Supply and Sanitation Programmes, PO Box 93190, 2509 AD The Hague, Netherlands.

International Union against Cancer, 3 Rue du Conseil General, 2105 Geneva, Switzerland.

MEDEX Group, University of Hawaii, 1833 Kalakaua Avenue, # 700, Honolulu, Hawaii, USA.

Teaching Aids at Low Cost (TALC), PO Box 49, St Albans, Herts AL1 4AX, UK.

UNICEF, 866 UN Plaza, United Nations, New York NY 10017, USA.

UNESCO, Unit for Cooperation with UNICEF and WFP, UNESCO, 7 Place de Fontenoy, 75700 Paris, France.

Water and Sanitation for Health Project (WASH), 1611 N. Kent Street (Room 1002), Arlington, Virginia 22209, USA.

World Health Organization, 1211 Geneva 27, Switzerland.

Index

approaches 18, 22
   definitions 16–17
Health Field Model 7
Health promotion 14–17
   communication in 18
   definition 15
   Ottawa Declaration 16–17
Health services 7–9, 11
HIV (Human Immunodeficiency
   Virus) *see* Acquired Immune
   Deficiency Syndrome
Honduras 63
Hong Kong 191
Horizontal planning 19, 22
Humour 52, 53
Hygiene 26, 27

IBFAN (International Baby Milk
   Action Network) 201
Illness behaviour *see* Behaviours
Immunization 39, 46, 140, 194
India 25, 130, 160, 173, 177, 196,
   204
   social inequalities 8, 16, 25,
     118, 122
Infectious diseases 4
Information Education and
   Communication (IEC) 17
Informed decision-making 18, 54
Innovations *see* Communication of
   Innovation Theory
Intersectoral collaboration 42, 126,
   194–6
Interviewing in research 216

Jamaica 173, 181
Job specifications
   project planning 225
   training 66

Kenya 183
Kwashiorkor 13

Laedza Batanani 132
Latin America *see* South America
Latrines *see* Water-related diseases
Lay workers 124–5
Leadership styles 104
Leaflets *see* Communication
Learning
   guidelines for effective 74
   types of 68–71

Learning aids 80
   films 82, 142
   flannelgraph 81–2
   flashcards 80
   flipcharts 80
   models 80
   overhead projector 83–4
   participatory 75, 124
   pictures 81
   slides 82
   video 82, 124
   wallcharts 80
Lesotho 142, 177
Lesson plan 85–6
Levels of intervention and influence
   14, 20, 43

Magazines 160
Malaria 137, 194
Malawi 134, 135, 199
Malnutrition 1, 13, 42, 135, 170,
   199
Management 225–6
Mass media 20, 54, 59, 61–2,
   145–67, 153–4
   media events 152
   media forums 154
   newspapers 148, 151–3
   print media 159–63
   radio 62, 149, 154–5
   television 145–9
Measles 4
Medicines 9, 12
Meetings *see* Groups
Mexico 131, 137, 190
Microphones for recording 158
Music *see* Popular media

Needs 117–18
   felt needs 117, 210
Nepal 58, 141
Networks *see* Social networks
Nigeria 31, 130, 137, 142, 147, 174
Non-governmental organisations
   (NGOs) 20, 21
Non-verbal communication *see*
   Communication
Norms 31; *see also* Social networks
Nutrition 42, 46, 193, 223

Objectives
   behavioural 73

Book list

* New in 1993.

Health Care Services
District Health Care: *R. Amonoo-Lartson, G. J. Ebrahim, H. J. Lovel, J. P. Ranken* – Intended for those involved in planning, administration and evaluation of health services at the district level.
Health Service Management: *edited by Kanani, Maneno and Schuter* – How to improve training by using workshops, with a modular approach.
Immunization in Practice: A practical training manual for health workers who give vaccines and for their trainers. In simple English it describes the process and how to carry out tasks.
My Name is Today: *D. Morley and H. Lovel* – Examines the economic, social, political, environmental and human causes of poor health in a clear and stimulating style. Also in French.
Partners in Evaluation: *M.-T. Feuerstein* – Basic principles of evaluation of any project or programme including management in community development, adult education etc. Also in Portuguese.
Primary Health Care; Reorienting Organisational Support: *Edited by G. J. Ebrahim and J. P. Rankin* – for students and teachers concerned with administrating, planning or delivering health services.
Primary Health Education: *Beverley Young* – How to teach health education in the classroom. Ideal for teachers and student teachers especially in primary schools.
* **Reaching Health for All:** *edited by J. Rohde, M. Chatterjee and D. Morley* – This book brings together 22 case studies from around the world to illustrate a wide range of approaches as well as problems in public health and development.
Rural Development; Putting the Last First: *Robert Chambers* – Describes why we all fail to reach the very poor and those who need help most.
Rural Water Supplies and Sanitation: *Peter Morgan* – A single, practical manual that will be invaluable to those working in the area of water supply and sanitation and associated health issues.
Sanitation Without Water: *Winblad, Kilama* – Practical information on how to design, build and operate compost and improved pit latrines.
* **Setting up Community Health Programmes:** *Ted Lankester* – A practical manual following a logical progression from before the programme starts through to running particular programmes and subsequent evaluation.

AIDS Education and Communication
The AIDS Handbook: *J. Hubley* – For those involved in AIDS education and community work, it covers origins, symptoms, transmission and counselling.
Preventing a Crisis; AIDS and Family Planning Work: *G. Gordon and A. Klouda* – Some up-to-date facts, ideas for integrating AIDS prevention into a health programme and approaches to prevention. Also in French and Arabic.
Talking AIDS: *G. Gordon and A. Klouda* – A practical handbook for community workers based on real questions and concerns voiced by people around the world. Also available in French and Arabic.

* **Strategies for Hope:** *Series editor Glen Williams* – A series of case study booklets and video programmes which aims to promote informed, positive thinking and practical action. No 1 From Fear to Hope. No 2 Living Positively With AIDS, No 3 AIDS Management, No 4 Meeting AIDS with Compassion, No 5 AIDS Orphans, No 6 The Caring Community, No 7 All Against AIDS. Booklets 1 to 6 also in French.

Mother and Child Care

Family Planning Clinic in Africa: *Richard and Judith Brown* – A new edition of this practical book for nurses, medical assistants and auxiliaries with information on setting up and running a contraception clinic.

Healthy Mothers, Happy Babies: *J. Hampton and J. Cleves Mosse* – Health problems in pregnancy and birth for mothers-to-be and community health workers.

Maternal and Child Health in Practice: *G. J. Ebrahim* – A complete course of training modules for middle level health workers.

Paediatric Practice in Developing Countries: *G. J. Ebrahim* – Intended for the District Officer who has to provide a comprehensive child care service for the district population.

Practical Care of Sick Children: *P. Dean and G. J. Ebrahim* – A practical handbook aimed at nurses, medical assistants and physicians, who have little or no training with sick children.

Primary Child Care Book One: *Maurice and Felicity King* – Comprehensive child care in simple language, well illustrated (see slide list for a matching slide set). Also in Portuguese.

* **State of the World's Children 1993:** *UNICEF* – Describes what it would take to meet the basic needs of all children.

A Village Struggles for Eye Health: *E. Sutter, A. Foster, V. Francis* – The story of Hanyane is an excellent primer for village community development using eye health as an example.

Where There is No Dentist: *Murray Dickson* – Excellent and well illustrated. Essential for all health workers who look into patients' mouths! Also in Portuguese.

Where There is No Doctor: *David Werner* – Highly practical, many illustrations. A must for those developing village programmes. Also in Arabic, Portuguese, Spanish, and an African edition in English. 'How to use Where There is no Doctor' is available in Portuguese only.

Nutrition and Child Growth

Helping Mothers to Breast Feed: *F. Savage King* – Up-to-date ideas about breast feeding, giving health workers practical guidance on how to prevent problems. Also in Arabic, French and Spanish.

Manual on Feeding Infants and Young Children: *Cameron and Hofvander* – A new edition completely re-written in 1990, simple and practical. Also in Spanish.

* **Nutrition for Developing Countries:** *F. Savage King and A. Burgess* – This new edition brings the subject up-to-date and to a slightly more advanced level, while retaining its simple approach.

Nutrition Handbook for Community Workers: *CFNI* – Working within the community to improve nutrition education.

Education and Communication

Child-to-child Readers: For teaching reading and about health simultaneously. 1. Dirty Water, 2. Good Food, 3. Accidents, 7. Not Just a cold, (Easy level 1 readers), 4. A Simple Cure, 5. Teaching Thomas, 6. Down with Fever, 8. Diseases Defeated, 9. Flies, 10. I Can Do It Too, (Level 2), 11. Deadly Habits (Level 3). Numbers 3, 4, 8 and 10, 'Le vieux roi et la petite fiancée', 'La fièvre du lion', 'L'Hyène aux Yeux de Poulet' and 'La Revanche de

Sanko-le-Lièvre' are available in French. Numbers 1 to 10 in Arabic and numbers 1 to 6 in Spanish.

Child-to-child Activity Sheets: Increasing pack size forces charge but a few sample sheets may be sent free on request.

* **Child-to-Child. A Resource Book:** *edited by G. Bonati and H. Hawes* – This book includes all the activity sheets, plus 'Approaches to Learning and Teaching', 'Doing it Better' and 'How to Run a Workshop'.

Facts for Life: *UNICEF* – A challenge to communicators of all kinds.

Health Care Together: *edited by M. Johnstone and S. Rifkin* – Training exercises for health workers in community based programmes. Designed to develop communication skills and teaching methods.

Health into Maths: Shows teachers in primary schools how to combine teaching health education and maths.

Helping Health Workers Learn: David Werner – Describing how to teach village health workers. Also in Portuguese and Spanish.

Puppets for Better Health: *Gill Gordon* – Now available at a much reduced price, this book shows how to make puppets, props and theatres and use them in teaching at community level.

Simple English is Better English: *Felicity Savage* – For those concerned with the need to communicate effectively; helps you to consider the English you use.

Teaching and Learning with Visual Aids: INTRAH – Covers the 'why, when and how' of visual aids with examples. For trainers generally.

Teaching Health-care Workers: *Fred Abbatt and Rosemary McMahon* – A simply written, well illustrated detailed guide for the teachers of health care workers.

Toys for Fun: *Edited by June Carlile* – A book of toys for pre-school children in English, French, Portuguese, Spanish, Swahili and Arabic all in one volume. Many illustrations.

Training Manual for Traditional Birth Attendants: *Compiled by Gill Gordon* – This book is a storehouse of facts and information which can be adapted to meet the needs of trainers and TBAs.

Disability and Appropriate Technology

* **Aches and Pains:** *J. Hampton* – A practical guide for sufferers, their families and health workers on the most common rheumatic diseases.

Alternative Limb Making: *AHRTAG* – The manufacture and fitting of low-cost below knee prostheses. Details of innovative products. Provides technical information and advice.

Disabled Village Children: *David Werner* – A guide for community health workers, rehabilitation workers, and families. A very comprehensive book. Also in French and Spanish.

How to Choose and Make a Cold Box: *AHRTAG* – Most appropriate cold boxes for vaccine transport in the area of those working in immunisation programmes.

How to Look after a Health Centre Store: *Battersby, AHRTAG* – A useful working guide on all aspects of storekeeping.

How to Look after a Refrigerator: *AHRTAG* – Revised edition including information on solar powered, as well as kerosene, gas and electric fridges. Also gives updated WHO guidelines.

* **How to make Simple Disability Aids:** *AHRTAG* – Many illustrations. Minimum text. A new revision of Simple Aids for Daily Living.

Insensitive Feet: *Leprosy Mission* – Management of foot problems in leprosy. (Free)

Personal Transport for Disabled People: *AHRTAG* – Designs for the local manufacture of wheelchairs, trolleys and tricycles from all over the world.

A Practical Guide to the Diagnosis and Treatment of Leprosy in the Basic Health Unit: *J. M. Watson* – An excellent booklet for the medical team and health worker. (Free)

We Can Play and Move: *AHRTAG* – From parent to expert, this book will help disabled children learn to move by playing with others. Well illustrated.

Medicine

Care of the Critically Ill Patient: *Wattes, Wilson, Leaver and Bagshawe* – A quick guide to the management of emergencies in hospitals and clinics.

⋆ **Clinical Tuberculosis:** *J. Crofton, N. Horne and F. Miller* – a practical, comprehensive and up-to-date guide to the diagnosis of all forms of tuberculosis in both adults and children. It includes sections on HIV infection in relation to tuberculosis.

Common Medical Problems in the Tropics: *C. R. Schull* – A comprehensive and practical handbook for medical and nursing staff, concentrating mainly on adult conditions. 419 pages packed with information.

Eye Diseases in Hot Climates: *John Sandford-Smith* – This second edition includes revisions on onchocerciasis, trachoma, eye examinations and the manifestation of AIDS.

Guidelines to Drug Usage: *G. Upunda, J. Yudkin and G. Brown* – A manual to assist in the rational purchase and prescription of drugs.

Medical Administration for Front-Line Doctors: *C. Andrew Pearson* – A practical guide to the management of district level hospitals, for money to maintenance and primary health care outreach.

Obstetric Emergencies: *J. Everett* – Presents the essential steps in the immediate management of the common obstetric problems.

Primary Anaesthesia: *edited by M. King* – A guide to the improvement of basic anaesthetic care, using safe, simple and cost effective methods.

Primary Surgery Vol. 1. Non-Trauma: *edited by M. King* – Release of pus, abdominal surgery, TB, leprosy, urology and much more besides.

Primary Surgery Vol. 2. Trauma: *edited by M. King* – An exhaustive account of all surgery procedures carried out in cases of injury.